AF614686

Bronchitis in Children - Latest Developments

Edited by Rada Markova

Published in London, United Kingdom

Bronchitis in Children - Latest Developments
http://dx.doi.org/10.5772/intechopen.101009
Edited by Rada Markova

Contributors
Terry W. Chin, Vyara Dimitrova, Asen Romanov Aleksiev, Penka Perenovska, Michiharu Shimosaka, Rada Markova, Clauden Louis, Latrice Johnson

First published in London, United Kingdom, 2024 by IntechOpen
IntechOpen is the global imprint of INTECHOPEN LIMITED, registered in England and Wales, registration number: 11086078, 5 Princes Gate Court, London, SW7 2QJ, United Kingdom

British Library Cataloguing-in-Publication Data
A catalogue record for this book is available from the British Library

Additional hard and PDF copies can be obtained from orders@intechopen.com

Bronchitis in Children - Latest Developments
Edited by Rada Markova
p. cm.
Print ISBN 978-1-83768-384-0
Online ISBN 978-1-83768-385-7
eBook (PDF) ISBN 978-1-83768-386-4

For EU product safety concerns:
IN TECH d.o.o., Prolaz Marije Krucifikse Kozulić 3, 51000 Rijeka, Croatia,
info@intechopen.com or visit our website at intechopen.com.

Meet the editor

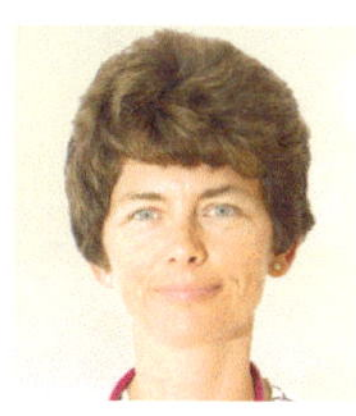

Assoc. Prof. Dr. Rada Markova graduated in medicine from the Medical University - Varna as the "Golden Hippocrates" of the graduating class. From the very beginning of her career, Dr. Rada Markova worked as a pediatrician in University Children's Clinics - initially in "St. Marina" UMHAT - Varna, and later - in the University Children's Hospital - Sofia, where she passed her rotating program in pediatrics, as a resident, assistant and senior assistant professor. She has experience in the Neonatology clinic- University Children's Hospital – Sofia and Intensive Care Unit of the same hospital. Over 17 years she worked as a pediatrician in the Pediatrics Clinic of UMHAT "Alexandrovska"- Sofia, Bulgaria. In 2004, Dr. Rada Markova obtained a specialty in pediatrics, in 2011 - in pediatric pulmonology. She has a master's degree in business administration and health management from UNWE- Sofia. In 2016 she completed her thesis on the topic: "Exhaled nitric oxide in children with bronchial asthma" and received the scientific title "doctor". In 2018 Dr. Markova became an Associate Professor in Pediatrics at Pleven Medical University- Bulgaria. Her scientific interests are in the field of general pediatrics and pediatric pulmonology - diagnosis and treatment of general pediatric conditions and problems, vaccine prophylaxis, children with infantile hemangiomas, effects and importance of air pollution for children's health, acute and chronic diseases of the respiratory system - bronchial asthma, cystic fibrosis, non-invasive methods of assessment of allergic airway inflammation, etc. She has specializations in the USA and Austria. In September 2012, she became the manager and conceptual founder of the biggest outpatient clinic in Sofia – "First Pediatric Consultative Clinic" - Sofia, part of Polyclinic Bulgaria. She devoted the following years of her life and work to ambulatory pediatrics, prevention in childhood and follow-up of children with chronic diseases. She has three children.

Contents

Preface IX

Chapter 1 1
Acute and Chronic Bronchitis in Childhood: Cystic Fibrosis
by Rada Markova

Chapter 2 17
Acute Bronchitis in Childhood
by Terry Chin

Chapter 3 35
Kinesitherapy and Ultrahigh-Frequency Current in Children with Bronchial Asthma
by Vyara Dimitrova, Assen Aleksiev and Penka Perenovska

Chapter 4 47
Advancements in Endobronchial Ultrasound
by Latrice Johnson and Clauden Louis

Chapter 5 61
A Case of Endotracheal Tube Damage during Maxillomandibular Osteotomy Found by Bronchofiberscope
by Michiharu Shimosaka

Preface

Acute bronchitis in childhood is one of the most common respiratory diseases. The disease affects all childhood age periods, being more severe in younger and premature children. It can be a reason for the development of respiratory failure and chronic lung pathology.

Despite advances in microbiological and virological diagnostics and therapy, the disease continues to be a diagnostic and therapeutic challenge.

The book describes the main etiological factors of acute and chronic bronchitis in childhood, the differences in the clinical symptoms and age characteristics in children. An important place is devoted to new therapeutic practices and preventive solutions.

The RSV - infection, the most severe viral infection in premature children, is covered as clinical symptoms, treatment, and prevention.

Cystic fibrosis, which is also the most common genetic disease involving the respiratory system, has been considered a common genetic cause of chronic - recurrent inflammation of the bronchi and the respiratory system.

An important place is devoted to the new methods of examination of the broncho-pulmonary system – endobronchial diagnostics.

A separate section is dedicated to kinesitherapy in respiratory diseases as the main non-pharmacological method to improve the clinical course of diseases.

The entire author team hopes to spark interest among our readers. We would appreciate your feedback and support!

With respect!

Dr. Rada Markova, M.D, Ph.D.
Associate Professor,
First Pediatric Consultative Clinic,
Sofia, Bulgaria

Medical University,
Pleven, Bulgaria

Chapter 1

Acute and Chronic Bronchitis in Childhood: Cystic Fibrosis

Rada Markova

Abstract

The chapter discusses the problems of clinical diagnosis, treatment, and follow-up of children with acute and chronic bronchitis. All clinical types of acute bronchitis are covered. Special focus is paid on cystic fibrosis—diagnosis, clinical features, and treatment. Affecting the lower respiratory tract (bronchi and bronchioles) is a very common phenomenon in childhood, most often with a viral etiology, sometimes bacterial, atypical, allergic, etc. Children's bronchi have a small amount of cartilaginous tissue, mainly smooth muscle tissue, and react to various triggers with bronchial spasm and increased mucus secretion. A significant part of pediatric pathology in early childhood is acute inflammatory diseases of the lower respiratory tract.

Keywords: acute bronchitis, chronic bronchitis, children, cystic fibrosis, clinical diagnosis

1. Introduction

Affecting the lower respiratory tract (bronchi and bronchioles) is a very common phenomenon in childhood, most often with viral etiology, sometimes bacterial, atypical, allergic, etc.

Children's bronchi have a small amount of cartilaginous tissue, mainly smooth muscle tissue, and react to various triggers with bronchial spasm and increased mucus secretion. A significant part of pediatric pathology in early childhood is acute inflammatory diseases of the lower respiratory tract.

2. *Acute bronchiolitis*

Acute bronchiolitis (AB) is a viral infectious disease of the lower respiratory tract that involves bronchioles (airways with a diameter of less than 2 mm) and is most often caused by respiratory syncytial virus (RSV) or human metapneumovirus (HMPV) [1–9], as well as by other viral agents [10–14]. It mainly affects ages 1–24 months, with an age prevalence between 3 and 6 months [15].

Acute bronchiolitis is the most common lower respiratory tract infection in the first year of life. There is an autumn-winter prevalence of the disease, which depends on the peak incidence of RSV, but is most often in the period from October to March [16, 17]. Boys get sick more often [18, 19].

There is still a high rate of hospitalization in these patients and a wide variability in clinical behavior and treatment approaches worldwide.

Children at increased risk of RSV infection or severe disease are [15]:

- Premature, low birth weight infants
- Groups with low socioeconomic status
- Parental smoking
- Broncho-pulmonary dysplasia as an underlying disease
- Severe congenital or acquired neurological diseases.
- Congenital heart defects with pulmonary hypertension
- Immune deficiencies
- Abnormalities of the respiratory tract
- Age under 3 months
- Hypotrophy, malabsorption, rickets

Acute bronchiolitis (AB), according to a WHO bulletin, has a significant impact on respiratory pathology worldwide with approximately 150 million cases per year, of which 7–13% are severe and require hospital treatment [15, 18, 19].

AB is essentially a self-limiting disease. Its treatment is supportive and includes oxygenation, adequate hydration, and temperature control. With early diagnosis and treatment, the prognosis is very good. The duration of the illness is usually 7–10 days, and most children recover without consequences. In some children, AB leads to recurrent "wheezing."

The clinical onset is most often atypical—irritability, decreased appetite, low temperature, and nasal discharge. In adults and in older children, RSV infection in 60% remains in the upper respiratory tract. After the incubation period of 2–5 days at a young age, RSV infection progressively affects the small airways with the development of cough, dyspnea, "wheezing," and difficulty feeding. Severe cases lead to manifestations of RDS with tachypnea, nasal breathing, dyspnea, and cyanosis [20].

The objective examination reveals tachypnea, expiratory dyspnea, tachycardia, fever, and diffuse "wheezing." Hypoxemia is the most accurate predictor of disease severity and correlates with the degree of tachypnea (over 50 bpm) [21].

Extrapulmonary manifestations include otitis media, myocarditis, arrhythmias, impaired secretion of ADH, etc. Acute bronchiolitis can be complicated by ARDS, bronchiolitis obliterans, congestive heart failure, myocarditis, secondary bacterial infection, and development of asthma [22–26]. Neurological complications with seizures and encephalopathy are rare.

Diagnosis of acute bronchiolitis is based on a well-taken history (most often patients with acute respiratory infections in the family), clinical presentation, the age of the child, the season of the disease, and the physical examination.

Laboratory studies tend to exclude other pathology. They include rapid RSV test from nasopharyngeal secretions, blood gas analysis or pulse oximetry, CBC, CRP, chest X-ray, etc. [27]. Usually, leukocytes are normal or slightly elevated with neutrophilia, which can be explained by a stress reaction [28].

X-ray of the lungs shows hyperinflation, and it is possible to observe lobular infiltrates, atelectasis, flat and low diaphragmatic cupola, and thickened bronchial walls. Atelectasis is a common finding and can cause arterial desaturation in these patients. An ECG is performed if there is evidence of arrhythmia or cardiomegaly from the lung X-ray [29, 30].

Pulse oximetry is an important method for determining the severity of AB and indications for hospital treatment. Patients with persistent TcSaO2 below 92% need hospital treatment and observation [31–33].

2.1 Treatment of acute bronchiolitis

The treatment of acute bronchiolitis is supportive, symptomatic, aiming rehydration and good oxygenation. The literature data on the issue of drug therapy in AB indicates very contradictory data. Only adequate oxygenation is surely effective and shortens the hospital stay [27, 30–32]. It can be performed with a nasal cannula, mask, tent, or mechanical ventilation.

The use of a bronchodilator has no proven effect and should be reserved only for patients with clinical improvement. It can be included orally or inhaled with a nebulizer or volume chamber [34, 35].

Regardless of their powerful anti-inflammatory effect and frequent application, corticosteroids (CS) do not lead to a significant improvement in the clinical status of patients and should be used only in severe cases [30, 36]. In cases of apnea, hypercapnia, and extreme hypoxemia, mechanical ventilation is required.

The application of oxygen—a helium mixture—Heliox is also important. In recent years, both in outpatient settings and as hospital treatment, the use of hypertonic 3% sodium chloride solution for the treatment of AB has been promoted as a safe, effective, and inexpensive way of treatment [37]. Chest physiotherapy is not recommended in the AB treatment plan.

Differences in therapeutic practices around the world are huge and lead in 2006 developing from the American Academy of Pediatrics (AAP) a *Consensus for behavior in acute Bronchiolitis* [30]:

- The diagnosis and the severity of the disease are determined by the clinical examination and history, not based on laboratory or imaging studies. Assessment of risk factors helps to decide for or against hospitalization.
- Bronchodilators should not be used routinely, but only when a clinical effect has been established [38].
- CS and antiviral medications should not be used routinely.
- Antibiotics are prescribed only when there is evidence of bacterial infection.
- Adequate hydration is very important.
- Oxygen therapy is carried out at oxygen saturation below 90% (or 92%).

- Palivizumab prophylaxis should only be used in certain groups.
- A very important element is the disinfection of staff's hands to prevent the transmission of infection in hospital wards.
- Parents should avoid smoking.
- Breastfeeding sick children is recommended.

After the implementation of the AAR recommendations in the USA, there was a decrease in hospitalizations (29%), length of stay (17%), RSV testing of nasopharyngeal swabs (52%), chest X-rays in AB in hospital, and outpatient cases [27, 30].

The criteria for hospitalization include [30]:

- Persistently measured oxygen saturation below 92% when breathing atmospheric air before beta 2 agonist administration.
- Significant tachypnea (>70–80 breaths/min)
- Expiratory dyspnea and intercostal retractions, signs of respiratory distress
- Desaturation when stopping the supply of 40% oxygen (3–4 L/min), cyanosis.
- Chronic lung disease
- Congenital cardiac malformation is especially associated with cyanosis and pulmonary hypertension.
- Prematurity
- Age under 3 months with an expected more severe course of the disease
- Impossible to perform oral rehydration in patients under 6 months of age.
- Difficulty feeding because of RDS.
- Social factor—parents who cannot take care of their children at home.

The prevention of RSV infection is essential for the general practitioner and for the narrow specialist—pulmonologist. Since 1967 attempts have been made to create and administer a formalin-inactivated RSV virus vaccine, still not been used for a massive vaccination. The use of the RSV-specific monoclonal antibody Palivizumab i.m. at a dose of 15 mg/kg/dose every 30 days from October to March significantly reduced the incidence of AB and the need for hospital treatment [39].

Acute bronchitis (AB) is an inflammatory disease of the large airways with a leading symptom—cough. In childhood, it is mainly associated with viral infections, most often descending upper respiratory airway infection, but it can be also connected to mechanical (dust, gas), chemical, or allergic inflammation of the respiratory tract. Clinically, it presents with a wet and productive cough with sputum discharge, sometimes with retrosternal pain when breathing or when coughing. It most often occurs as a self-limiting disease with complete recovery in 7–14 days (maximum 28 days) [15, 18].

Chronic bronchitis is defined as a recurrent inflammation and degeneration of the bronchial wall. In chronic bronchitis, increased mucus production is observed either due to increased secretion or due to impaired clearance. Defining chronic bronchitis in childhood, as well as its distribution, is very difficult due to overlapping clinical diagnoses.

For adults, it is defined as diffuse and non-specific inflammation of the bronchi, manifestation of cough, and daily expectoration within 3 months for 2 consecutive years. Some authors apply this definition to children as well or define chronic bronchitis as a productive cough lasting more than 4 weeks regardless of treatment, with expectoration and an auscultation finding of wheezing and variable wet crackles bilaterally.

2.2 Etiology

Acute bronchitis (AB) has a viral etiology in 90%, and a bacterial etiology in 10%, rarely others. Viral agents include adenoviruses, influenza, parainfluenza, rhinovirus, RSV, coxsackievirus, HSV, etc. Secondary bacterial infection can be observed from Str. pneumoniae, *M. catarrhalis*, *Chlamydia pneumonia*, *H. influenzae*, *M. pneumoniae* [40]. Both active and passive smoking can increase the risk of recurrent bronchitis. Less common causes are GERD, fungal infections, etc. The seasonal prevalence of acute bronchitis is mainly during autumn and winter season.

- Pathoanatomic forms: catarrhal, fibrinous, purulent, and necrotizing.
- By localization of the inflammatory process: diffuse or limited.
- By course: primary or secondary (within another disease)
- According to the presence or absence of bronchospasm: obstructive or non-obstructive

The clinical course could be:

2.2.1 Acute bronchitis, acute tracheobronchitis

It is defined as an inflammation of the epithelium of the trachea and large and medium bronchi. It appears with a preserved general condition, normal or low-grade temperature, and cough, which can be mainly dry, painful (typical for tracheitis), or wet with expectoration.

Physically, diminished or more aggravated vesicular breathing with/without dry wheezing sounds, and large and medium wet crackles, often of a transient nature is found.

Normal laboratory values are observed, lung X-ray is not necessary—if done it is normal or shows thickened pulmonary roots and peribronchial changes [29].

It passes with symptomatic therapy for 8–10 days, which includes a home regime, mucolytics, inhalations, antipyretic when needed, and very rarely the inclusion of antibiotic treatment.

2.2.2 Bronchitis obstructiva, asthmatiformis

It is most often caused by RSV, Parainfluenzavirus, etc. It starts as an upper respiratory tract infection and gradually develops tachypnea, expiratory dyspnea, nasal breathing, etc.

Physically, a hypersonic percussive tone is observed, diminished vesicular breathing with prolonged expiration, and dry wheezing noises bilaterally are established.

Pulmonography demonstrates evidence of hyperinflation of the lung parenchyma—emphysema [29]. Laboratory parameters are normal, and eosinophilia is possible. The treatment is the same as for acute bronchitis with the addition of bronchodilators, with/without corticosteroids [27].

- Bronchiolitis acuta (see above)

- Bronchiolitis obliterans

Acute bronchiolitis, even with a protracted course, improves in 2 weeks. If the symptoms of respiratory failure, obstruction, and hypoxemia persist, the development of bronchiolitis obliterans is possible.

Radiologically, it is demonstrated with ultra-transparency of the lung parenchyma, reduced vascular pattern, peribronchial thickening, and the development of bronchiectasis [29].

Etiologically, it is most often associated with adenovirus, influenza virus, and mycoplasma infection, but not with RSV [10, 11]. It leads to the development of chronic respiratory failure and cor pulmonale.

A rare form, but potentially fatal, is the so-called *plastic bronchitis*—the formation of solid casts of the tracheobronchial tree. For unexplained reasons, this type of bronchitis is seen more often in patients with congenital cardiac defects and Fontan operations. It is believed that pathogenetically this bronchitis is associated with high thoracic lymphatic pressure.

Acute and chronic bronchitis are the main reason for a doctor's consultation on a global aspect, and their probable incidence is about 20% in school age. In acute bronchitis, gender dependence is not established, in chronic bronchitis the male gender is prevalent.

2.2.3 Bronchitis chronica (chronic bronchitis)

According to the definition of WHO: "chronic bronchitis is a diffuse and non-specific inflammation of the bronchi, which is manifested by cough and mucopurulent expectoration with autumn-winter seasonality for at least 3 months in two or three consecutive years."

About 2–3 times more often affects the male sex, more typical for smokers (5×), and increases in frequency with age [15, 18, 19].

Chronic inflammation occurs due to the disruption of natural defense mechanisms, the damaging role of exogenous factors: moisture, dust, cold, steam, gases, smoking, etc., in combination with endogenous factors (kyphoscoliosis, diabetes, heart failure, immune deficiency, etc.)

Pathogenetically, there is chronic hypoxemia, which leads to an increase in pulmonary vascular resistance, metabolic acidosis, and polycythemia, followed by the development of cor pulmonale and pulmonary hypertension.

Pathoanatomically, hyperemia is found, as well as edema, and lymphocytic infiltration of the bronchial wall, followed by mucosal atrophy, and reduction of secretory glands and elastic fibers.

The clinic is represented by three main symptoms:

- Cough
- Expectoration—mucopurulent
- Shortness of breath, with/without chest or abdominal pain

Physically, sonorous, or hyper sonorous percussive tone is found, reduced respiratory mobility, and diffuse dry crackles are detected.

Pulmonography shows low standing of the diaphragmatic cupola, the presence of pulmonary emphysema, and fibrosis [29].

Chronic bronchitis occurs with episodes of exacerbation and remission. Complications include recurrent pneumonias, bronchiectasis, pulmonary emphysema and COPD, and the development of cor pulmonale.

In terms of differential diagnosis, the following are discussed: cystic fibrosis, asthma, PCD, TB, foreign body in the respiratory tract, aspiration, immune deficiency, etc.

In periods of exacerbation, antibiotic treatment is carried out according to the antibiogram of the pathogenic flora from sputum (throat secretion), secretolytic, and bronchodilator therapy [34, 35]. Physiotherapy—postural drainage, ultrasound of the chest, and magnetotherapy are also widely used.

Recurrent episodes of acute and chronic bronchitis are atypical for childhood and should prompt the pediatrician to look for childhood asthma. In such children, the presence of family burden and personal atopic characteristics increases the risk of childhood asthma [21–26].

The presence of recurrent bronchitis points to the search for immune deficiency—IgA or IgG transient or subclasses.

In addition to chronic bronchitis, one of the most common reasons for chronic bronchitis in childhood is cystic fibrosis.

Cystic fibrosis (CF) is the most common genetic multisystem disease affecting Caucasians with autosomal recessive inheritance. The disease has an average incidence among Caucasians of 1 in 2000 to 2500 live births. The carrier frequency is 4–5% in the population [41, 42].

The cystic fibrosis gene is located on the long arm of the 7th chromosome, locus 7q31.2, and was mapped in 1989. The cystic fibrosis protein called cystic fibrosis transmembrane conductance regulator (CFTR) is a transmembrane transport protein with a complex configuration [43]. More than 1600 mutations in the CFTR gene are currently known, of which delta F508 is the most common. Mutations are divided into 6 classes [42, 44].

CF is a congenital genetic disease. The phenotype manifestation of the disease can begin at different ages. As a rule, class I and class II mutations cause earlier and more severe clinical symptoms, while those of the other classes underlie milder cases [43]. The phenotype–genotype correlation is more demonstrative for symptoms from the digestive and reproductive systems and less pronounced for pulmonary manifestations [45].

Clinical diagnosis: In 5–10% of children with CF, presentation is in the neonatal period with meconium ileus. This is a reason for early diagnosis of the disease. Sick children are born with healthy lungs.

Typical *neonatal and infant clinical manifestations* of the disease include cough with different characteristics—dry or more moist and productive, sometimes—pertussis-like with painful expectoration, manifestations of bronchospasm with difficulty resolved bronchial obstruction by conventional treatment, recurrent broncho-pulmonary infections in infancy with frequent detection of *S. aures* from throat secretions (or sputum).

In this period, manifestations of GER, cholestatic jaundice, chronic diarrhea with malabsorption, bulky and greasy stools, and lack of weight gain are common. The last symptom is of leading importance in infancy for an active search for the diagnosis. Infants have a preserved, even increased appetite, in the absence of weight gain. The "salty kiss" symptom is also positive in infancy. A special clinical form characterized by generalized hypoproteinemic edema and anemic syndrome is the so-called edematous-anemic form of the disease, which is observed mainly in the age up to 1 year [45, 46].

In *early childhood*, the clinical symptoms are presented with: chronic cough with/without sputum discharge, recurrent infections of the respiratory tract, colonization with a wider range of microorganisms: *S. aureus*, *H. influenzae*, *Pseudomonas aeruginoza*, *S. maltofila*, etc., chronic diarrhea, manifestations of hypovitaminosis for fat-soluble vitamins. Manifestations of rectal prolapse and distal intestinal pseudo-obstruction syndrome (DIOS) are more common. Initial bronchiectasis is detected more often in chest X-rays in patients with more marked pulmonary symptoms. Changes begin on the nails and fingers with clubbing and "drumstick" nail types. At this age, changes in the rheology of the bile also occur—"thick bile syndrome" with possible gall bladder calculus and hepatic steatosis. During the summer months, electrolyte disturbances and a tendency to dehydration are observed [45, 46].

At school age, the manifestations of chronic respiratory failure dominate with changes in the chest, which becomes emphysematous with an increased anterior–posterior diameter. The auscultation phenomena are most often represented by a hypersonic percussion tone, weakened vesicular breathing with a rich exudative finding of moist rhonchi and crepitations, maybe a localized finding of lung inflammation or bronchiectasis, broncho-obstructive symptoms are also common.

With the development of pulmonary hypertension, ECG changes and accentuated cardiac T2 may be detected [45, 46].

At this age, colonization with *Pseudomonas aeruginosa* (PA) is of leading importance for the evolution of the disease. When it is first established, an eradication course is recommended. In chronic PA infection, pulmonary exacerbations are treated. Pulmonary complications are observed: atelectasis, bronchiectasis, pneumothorax, pulmonary bleeding, etc. With poor therapeutic control of the disease, children have an asthenic and cachectic appearance, and reduced subcutaneous fat tissue. It is not uncommon to involve the upper respiratory tract with the development of chronic rhinosinusitis and nasal polyposis. It is the cause of difficult nasal breathing and bacterial colonization of nasal secretions by *Staphylococcus aureus*. Advanced involvement of the endocrine pancreas leads to manifestations of diabetes mellitus, which necessitates additional insulin treatment. Changes in bone density are observed with the development of osteoporosis. In puberty, mental and emotional problems intensify, which complicate the treatment of the disease.

In patients of *reproductive age*, reduced fertility in women and azoospermia and sterility in men have been observed.

Laboratory diagnosis of the disease has several steps:

A. Related to the diagnosis of the disease:

- Possible performance of neonatal screening—carried out in some countries—USA, Australia, some European countries—immunoreactive trypsinogen is examined and only in case of deviation a sweat test is carried out.

- Sweat test—"gold standard"—positive result above 60 mmol/l (mEq/l), at least 2 positive tests are required, in 1% of patients the sweat test is normal.

- Fecal elastase 1, steatorrhea, coprocitogramm

- Genetic DNA analysis with determination of the type of mutation, prenatal diagnosis in the case of another pregnancy in the family

- Determination of nasal or rectal transepithelial potential difference (NTP)

B. Related to monitoring of diagnosed patients:

- Blood gas analysis demonstrating metabolic alkalosis, hypoxemia with/without hypercapnia

- Changes in electrolytes—hypochloremia, hyponatremia

- Determination of the fraction of exhaled nitric oxide (FeNO)—(reduced in patients with CF)

- Carrying out pulmonary function test (PFT)—most often indicates a mixed ventilatory defect with a reduction of VC and dynamic indicators

- Chest X-ray depending on the involvement of the lung, can demonstrate a very rich image "picture," in the terminal stages we talk about the so-called "honeycomb": pulmonary emphysema and fibrosis, bronchiectasis, sites of old and fresh inflammatory changes, asthenic chest, prominent arch of the pulmonary artery, possible atelectasis, etc. [41, 42].

- Liver enzymes—most often they are increased with a dominant change in cholestatic indicators, coagulation factors, total protein and serum albumins also change dynamically.

- Blood analysis: accelerated ESR, leukocytosis and neutrophilia in bacterial infection, data on hemoconcentration in dehydration and chronic hypoxemia

- Abdominal ultrasound

- Blood glucose, blood glucose profile, oral glucose tolerance test—OGTT

- Wrist X-ray for assessing the bone age

2.3 Follow-up of CF patients

CF is currently an incurable disease. In recent decades, a significant improvement in the duration and quality of life of these patients has been observed. The effect of therapy is complex and is based on self-control and training of patients, close cooperation with a team of professionals, new medications and recommendations for treatment [47].

Around the world, the monitoring and control of these patients is most often carried out in the so-called "Cystic Fibrosis Centers" (CFCs), most of which are affiliated with university hospitals or outpatient follow-up clinics. CFCs teams include a pulmonologist, gastroenterologist, nutritionist, physical therapist, social worker, psychologist, trained nurses, microbiologist, and more.

In outpatient care (outpatient care): patients are followed up every 1–3 months, and newly diagnosed patients—every month. Each visit includes a routine physical examination, measurement of height, weight, BMI, pulse oximetry, functional respiratory testing, and microbiological analysis of sputum or deep throat secretions. At each visit, the treatment plan and any changes to it are discussed in detail. Patients with positive *P. aeruginosa* or *B. cepacia* must be separated from the others [47].

In case of in-patient care, beds are provided for immediate admission, separate rooms for 1 child each, and strict control of infectious transmission is observed—hand hygiene, use of disinfectants, and clear antibiotic treatment protocols. Smooth transition into the age of 16–18 years from a pediatric team to a team of internists.

A CF patient's annual protocol includes the following:

- History of events since the last examination, previous illnesses, and treatment.
- Immunizations, annual flu vaccine.
- Detailed clinical examination: anthropometric data: height, weight, head circumference, BMI, growth curves
- Review by a physiotherapist of drainage techniques used, frequency of sessions, and use of respiratory therapy (bronchodilators, nebulized antibiotics, rhDNase). Overview of inhaler used and cleaning technique.
- Spirometry in patients older than 5 years.
- Dietary reassessment and commentary on diet, knowledge and dosage of pancreatic enzymes, vitamin therapy, additional calorie foods
- Time to work with a social worker and a psychologist
- Blood collection for: CBC and smear, C-reactive protein, IgG, serum electrolytes, blood glucose, kidney and liver samples, fat-soluble vitamins: A, D, E, K, prothrombin time, IgE, antibodies against *Aspergillus fumigatus*—RAST or skin test, antibodies against *P. aeruginosa*
- Fecal test for pancreatic elastase 1, steatorrhea
- X-ray of the lungs, abdominal ultrasound, microbiology of sputum/deep throat secretion [47].

2.4 Treatment of patients with CF

Outpatient treatment for children with cystic fibrosis has several aspects:

Regarding nutrition and pancreatic replacement therapy: recommendations for 3 main meals, intermediate meals [18, 19], intake of more salt in the summer months, fluids, intake of high-calorie food, fat-soluble vitamins (Aquadeks), pancreatic enzymes—Kreon 25,000 E (dose 500–2000 E lipase/kg/dose at the beginning of the meal, without disturbing the integrity of the microsomes in the capsules). The main criterion for enzyme sufficiency is weight gain and the number of bowel movements per day. Good nutritional status is directly related to FEV1 and lung function in children with CF. There are affordable caloric foods: Fresubin, Nutrinidrink, and Infatrini, which help weight gain in case of malnutrition.

Regarding the lung, the therapy is inhaled, antibiotic, mucolytic, and enzymatic.

Inhalation therapy consists of daily inhalations with 0.9% sodium chloride and hypertonic sodium chloride solution—1.5%, 3%, 4.5–7%. The side effect of hypertonic solutions could be possibly bronchospasm. Mannitol is also inhaled in some countries. The aim is to facilitate secretions and improve mucociliary clearance.

Mucolytics—Mistabron, N-Acetylcystein, Fluimucil, are mainly administered orally, and the dose is increased in case of pulmonary exacerbation.

Enzyme therapy: Pulmozyme/Rh-Dornase Alpha/—recombinant human deoxyribonuclease (rhDNase). It is administered by inhalation 1× daily (1 ampule of 2 ml, 2500E/, from 5 years of age.

Prophylactic long-term treatment with inhaled antibiotics when chronic P. aeruginosa infection is proven—TOBI 300 mg/5 ml 2×/day, 1 amp each, Arikase 1×/day, Colistin 2000000E 2×/day, etc. They are applied with aerosol inhalers or powder inhalers, 1-2×/day in cycles of 28 days on, 28 days off. Their role is to suppress chronic pseudomonas infection and improve lung function.

Pulmonary exacerbations usually require hospital treatment and parenteral administration of combinations of broad-spectrum antibiotics according to an antibiogram in maximum dosage and maximum duration of 14–21 days. Oral courses with combined penicillins, cephalosporins, macrolides, and quinolones are administered in outpatient settings [48].

- *Physiotherapy*—daily, parents are trained in various techniques—mechanical percussion, postural bronchial drainage, autogenous drainage, breathing with a flutter, breathing against positive expiratory pressure (PEP mask), breathing with oral high-frequency oscillation, the so-called vest—device, etc.

- *Gene therapy and CFTR modifiers*—this is a therapy of the future for CF, there are many studies proving a good effect of the latter in some mutations, still with a high economic cost.

- *Lung transplantation*—the last choice for the so-called end–stage CF – has more experience in the USA, and few transplant centers in Europe.

The future is open to new therapeutic methods for children with CF, for the last decades, the life expectancy for most countries has increased many times. The result of the treatment is a complex of measures and methods concerning training, self-control, nutrition, physiotherapy, and inhalation therapy, to be well monitored by qualified specialists in this serious disease [46].

Author details

Rada Markova[1,2]

1 First Pediatric Consultative Clinic, Sofia, Bulgaria

2 Medical University, Pleven, Bulgaria

*Address all correspondence to: rada_markova@yahoo.com

References

[1] Bosis S, Esposito S, Niesters HG, Crovari P, Osterhaus AD, Principi N. Impact of human metapneumovirus in childhood: Comparison with respiratory syncytial virus and influenza viruses. Journal of Medical Virology. 2005;**75**(1):101-104

[2] Caracciolo S, Minini C, Colombrita D, Rossi D, Miglietti N, Vettore E. Human metapneumovirus infection in young children hospitalized with acute respiratory tract disease: Virologic and clinical features. The Pediatric Infectious Disease Journal. 2008;**27**(5):406-412

[3] Risnes KR, Radtke A, Nordbø SA, Grammeltvedt AT, Døllner H. Human metapneumovirus--occurrence and clinical significance. Tidsskrift for den Norske Lægeforening. 2005;**125**(20):2769-2772

[4] Werno AM, Anderson TP, Jennings LC, Jackson PM, Murdoch DR. Human metapneumovirus in children with bronchiolitis or pneumonia in New Zealand. Journal of Paediatrics and Child Health. 2004;**40**(9-10):549-551

[5] Garcia-Garcia ML, Calvo C, Casas I, et al. Human metapneumovirus bronchiolitis in infancy is an important risk factor for asthma at age 5. Pediatric Pulmonology. 2007;**42**(5):458-464

[6] Dollner H, Risnes K, Radtke A, Nordbo SA. Outbreak of human metapneumovirus infection in norwegian children. The Pediatric Infectious Disease Journal. 2004;**23**(5):436-440

[7] Garcia ML, Calvo Rey C, Martin del Valle F, et al. Respiratory infections due to metapneumovirus in hospitalized infants. Anales de Pediatría (Barcelona, Spain). 2004;**61**(3):213-218

[8] McNamara PS, Flanagan BF, Smyth RL, Hart CA. Impact of human metapneumovirus and respiratory syncytial virus co-infection in severe bronchiolitis. Pediatric Pulmonology. 2007;**42**(8):740-743

[9] Semple MG, Cowell A, Dove W, et al. Dual infection of infants by human metapneumovirus and human respiratory syncytial virus is strongly associated with severe bronchiolitis. The Journal of Infectious Diseases. 2005;**191**(3):382-386

[10] Counihan ME, Shay DK, Holman RC, Lowther SA, Anderson LJ. Human parainfluenza virus-associated hospitalizations among children less than five years of age in the United States. The Pediatric Infectious Disease Journal. 2001;**20**(7):646-653

[11] Mansbach JM, McAdam AJ, Clark S, Hain PD, Flood RG, Acholonu U. Prospective multicenter study of the viral etiology of bronchiolitis in the emergency department. Academic Emergency Medicine. 2008;**15**(2): 111-118

[12] Williams JV, Harris PA, Tollefson SJ, Halburnt-Rush LL, Pingsterhaus JM, Edwards KM. Human metapneumovirus and lower respiratory tract disease in otherwise healthy infants and children. The New England Journal of Medicine. 2004;**350**(5):443-450

[13] Arnold JC, Singh KK, Spector SA, Sawyer MH. Human bocavirus: Prevalence and clinical spectrum at a children's hospital. Clinical Infectious Diseases. 2006;**43**(3):283-288

[14] Meissner HC. Selected populations at increased risk from respiratory syncytial viral infection. Pediatric Infectious Disease. 2003;**22**:S40

[15] Barclay L. AAP Updates Guidelines on Bronchiolitis in Young Children. Medscape: Medical News. 27 Oct 2014. Available from: http://www.medscape.com/viewarticle/833884; [Accessed: November 1, 2014]

[16] Fodha I, Vabret A, Ghedira L, et al. Respiratory syncytial virus infections in hospitalized infants: Association between viral load, virus subgroup, and disease severity. Journal of Medical Virology. 2007;**79**(12):1951-1958

[17] McConnochie KM, Hall CB, Walsh EE, Roghmann KJ. Variation in severity of respiratory syncytial virus infections with subtype. The Journal of Pediatrics. 1990;**117**(1 Pt 1):52-62

[18] Ralston SL, Lieberthal AS, Meissner HC, Alverson BK, Baley JE, Gadomski AM, et al. Clinical practice guideline: The diagnosis, management, and prevention of bronchiolitis. Pediatrics. 27 Oct 2014;**134**(5):e1474-e1502

[19] American Academy of Pediatrics. Subcommittee on diagnosis and management of acute bronchiolitis. [Guideline] Diagnosis and management of bronchiolitis. Pediatrics. Oct 2006;**118**(4):1774-1793

[20] Tristram DA, Welliver RC. Bronchiolitis. In: Long SS, Pickering LK, Prober CG, editors. Principles and Practice of Pediatric Infectious Diseases. 2nd ed. New York: Churchill Livingstone; 2003. p. 213

[21] Brand PL, Baraldi E, Bisgaard H. Definition, assessment and treatment of wheezing disorders in preschool children: An evidence-based approach. The European Respiratory Journal. 2008;**32**(4):1096-1110

[22] Castro-Rodríguez JA, Holberg CJ. A clinical index to define risk of asthma in young children with recurrent wheezing. American Journal of Respiratory and Critical Care Medicine. 2000;**162**:1403-1406

[23] Martinez FD, Wright AL. Asthma and wheezing in the first six years of life. The group health medical associates. The New England Journal of Medicine. 1995;**332**(3):133-138

[24] Guilbert TW, Morgan WJ. Atopic characteristics of children with recurrent wheezing at high risk for the development of childhood asthma. The Journal of Allergy and Clinical Immunology. 2004;**114**(6):1282-1287

[25] Henderson J, Granell R. Associations of wheezing phenotypes in the first 6 years of life with atopy, lung function and airway responsiveness in mid-childhood. Thorax. 2008;**63**(11):974-980. DOI: 10.1136/thx.2007.093187

[26] Bacharier LB, Boner A, Carlsen KH. Diagnosis and treatment of asthma in childhood: A PRACTALL consensus report. European Pediatric Asthma Group. Allergy. 2008;**63**(1):5-34

[27] Shaw KN, Bell LM, Sherman NH. Outpatient assessment of infants with bronchiolitis. American Journal of Diseases of Children. 1991;**145**:151-155

[28] Marguet C, Bocquel N, Benichou J, et al. Neutrophil but not eosinophil inflammation is related to the severity of a first acute epidemic bronchiolitis in young infants. Pediatric Allergy and Immunology. 2008;**19**(2):157-165

[29] Bada C, Carreazo NY, Chalco JP, Huicho L. Inter-observer agreement in interpreting chest X-rays on children with acute lower respiratory tract infections and concurrent wheezing. São Paulo Medical Journal. 2007;**125**(3):150-154

[30] Perlstein PH, Kotagal UR, Bolling C, et al. Evaluation of an evidence-based guideline for bronchiolitis. Pediatrics. 1999;**104**(6):1334-1341

[31] Unger S, Cunningham S. Effect of oxygen supplementation on length of stay for infants hospitalized with acute viral bronchiolitis. Pediatrics. 2008;**121**(3):470-475

[32] AHRQ Publication Number 03-E009, January 2003. Agency for Healthcare Research and Quality, Rockville, MD. Management of Bronchiolitis in Infants and Children. Summary, Evidence Report/Technology Assessment: Number 69. US Department of Health and Human Services. Available from: http://www.ahrq.gov/clinic/epcsums/broncsum.htm [Accessed: February 28, 2010]

[33] Dornelles CT, Piva JP, Marostica PJ. Nutritional status, breastfeeding, and evolution of infants with acute viral bronchiolitis. Journal of Health, Population, and Nutrition. 2007;**25**(3):336-343

[34] Kellner JD, Ohlsson A, Gadomski AM, Wang EE. Efficacy of bronchodilator therapy in bronchiolitis. A meta-analysis. Archives of Pediatrics & Adolescent Medicine. 1996;**150**(11):1166-1172

[35] Dobson JV, Stephens-Groff SM, McMahon SR, Stemmler MM, Brallier SL, Bay C. The use of albuterol in hospitalized infants with bronchiolitis. Pediatrics. 1998;**101**(3 Pt 1):361-368

[36] Leer JA Jr, Green JL, Heimlich EM, Hyde JS, Moffet HL, Young GA. Corticosteroid treatment in bronchiolitis. A controlled, collaborative study in 297 infants and children. American Journal of Diseases of Children. 1969;**117**(5):495-503

[37] Kuzik BA, Al-Qadhi SA, Kent S, et al. Nebulized hypertonic saline in the treatment of viral bronchiolitis in infants. The Journal of Pediatrics. 2007;**151**(3):266-270 270.e1

[38] Flores G, Horwitz RI. Efficacy of beta2-agonists in bronchiolitis: A reappraisal and meta-analysis. Pediatrics. 1997;**100**(2 Pt 1):233-239

[39] Wegner S, Vann JJ, Liu G, Byrns P, Cypra C, Campbell W. Direct cost analyses of palivizumab treatment in a cohort of at-risk children: Evidence from the North Carolina Medicaid program. Pediatrics. 2004;**114**(6):1612-1619

[40] McNamara PS, Flanagan BF, Baldwin LM, et al. Interleukin 9 production in the lungs of infants with severe respiratory syncytial virus bronchiolitis. Lancet. 2004;**363**(9414):1031-1037

[41] Behrman. Cystic fibrosis. In: Nelson Textbook of Pediatrics. W.B. Sounders Company;

[42] Hodson M, Bush A, Geddes D. Cystic Fibrosis. 2007

[43] Struyvenberg MR, Martin CR, Steven D. FreedmanJ-Exocrine pancreatic insufficiency. BMC Medicine. 2007:**15**;29

[44] Cystic fibrosis. In: Kendig's Disorders of the Respiratory Tract in Children. Sixth ed. pp. 838-883

[45] Petersen NT, Høiby N, Mordhorst CH, Lind K, Flensborg EW, Bruun B. Respiratory infections in cystic fibrosis patients caused by virus, chlamydia and mycoplasma—possible synergism with Pseudomonas aeruginosa. Acta Paediatrica Scandinavica. Sep 1981;**70**(5):623-628. DOI: 10.1111/j.1651-2227

[46] Conwey SP, Brownlee CG, Peckham DK. Antibiotic treatment of multidrug-resistant organisms in cystic fibrosis. American Journal of Respiratory and Critical Care Medicine. 2003;**2**(4):321-332

[47] Kerem E, Conway S, Elborn S, et al. For the Consensus Committee: Standards of care for patients with cystic fibrosis: A European consensus. Journal of Cystic Fibrosis. 2005;**4**:7-26

[48] Flume P, Mogayzel P Jr, Robinson K, et al. Cystic fibrosis pulmonary guidelines: Pulmonary complications: Hemoptysis and pneumothorax. American Journal of Respiratory and Critical Care Medicine. 2010;**0**:201002-0157OCv1. Available from: http://ajrccm.atsjournals.org

Chapter 2

Acute Bronchitis in Childhood

Terry Chin

Abstract

There will be a discussion of the manifestation of acute bronchitis in children and note differences with that seen in the adult population. In particular, the need for identifying the specific cause of coughing such as inhalation of a foreign body or diagnosing the newly recognized protracted bacterial bronchitis (PBB) in children is emphasized. Understanding the differing pathophysiology of afferent hypersensitivity and inflammatory infiltrates in the bronchial epithelium enables for different therapeutic approaches. Therefore, the chapter concludes with a discussion on the role for anti-inflammatory and antimicrobial therapies in children, as well as possible intervention to the neuronal hypersensitivity. Anti-tussive and mucolytic modes of treatment are also reviewed.

Keywords: acute bronchitis, protracted bacterial bronchitis, acute cough, chronic cough, children

1. Introduction

The inflammatory response in the lung protects the person from microorganisms or particles which may reach the airway surface. It augments other host defense mechanisms such as mucociliary clearance, defensins, and immunoglobulins. If the response is inadequate to eradicate offending substances, the subsequent inflammatory process can damage lung tissue in addition to any direct toxic or deleterious effects by the infectious organisms or particles. Also, if the immune response is excessive or poorly-regulated, the subsequent inflammation can be destructive to lung tissue and contribute to chronic lung disease.

Technically, the term "bronchitis" indicates inflammation of the bronchial tubes. However, functionally, the presence of coughing can indicate bronchial inflammation and therefore most reviews of acute and chronic bronchitis are actually discussions of acute and chronic coughing. Coughing is the body's effort to clear the airways of mucus or any foreign substances which may be present in bronchial tubes. As such, it augments the body's mucociliary clearance mechanism. As a symptom, coughing is one of the most frequent reasons for seeking medical attention and intervention in children worldwide. Therefore there are socioeconomic implications and consequences for the patient and patient's family as well as the health care system and society in general. However, this paper will examine the practitioner's approach in evaluating and managing these patients with attention to the various pathogenic mechanisms which may be involved.

Although it is uniformly accepted that chronic cough in adults is defined as coughing lasting greater than 8 weeks, there is some ambiguity for children. The American College of Chest Physicians (ACCP) through its CHEST Expert Cough Panel and the European Respiratory Society (ERS) both defined chronic cough in children as coughing greater than 4 weeks in duration [1, 2]. Acute coughing is further defined to last less than 2 weeks and subacute cough 2–4 weeks. In contrast, the British Thoracic Society (BTS) defined acute cough in children as lasting for less than 3 weeks, subacute coughing lasting 3–8 weeks and chronic coughing persisting greater than 8 weeks [3]. These time periods have also been adopted by two Asian groups, the Japanese Respiratory and Chinese Thoracic Societies but there is no distinction between adults and children [4, 5]. Western guidelines emphasized the need to separate the two age groups [1, 2]. A recent systematic review and meta-analysis of chronic cough in China utilized the 4 week duration as the cut-off [6]. The ACCP guidelines state that for patients greater than 14 years of age the approach to evaluation and management is similar to their guidelines for the adult [7].

This chapter will discuss acute bronchitis in children since chronic bronchitis is a topic presented elsewhere. Since there is some ambiguity as to its duration, coughing between 2 and 8 weeks (subacute bronchitis) will also be mentioned.

2. Children are not little adults

Although anatomic differences are minimal between adults and those greater than 14 years old, there are important differences in infants and especially in neonates and need to be considered. Anatomic differences in airway morphology such as total surface area dimension to weight between neonates and adults result in a much higher vulnerability or susceptibility of the child's airway surfaces to noxious or toxic insults, such as air pollution [8]. Children have a higher respiratory rate than adults and therefore inhale more air relative to their size than do adults. Additionally, they tend to spend more time outdoors, playing and being active. Therefore, they are exposed more often and to a greater degree to polluted outdoor air than adults. There is an association between particulate air pollution with acute bronchitis in children and rates of bronchitis decrease in areas in which the particulate concentration has declined [9]. This correlation has been further supported by a recent review of 34 studies, 16 of which were subjected to meta-analysis [10]. Another investigation indicated a possible role of low ambient temperature interacting with the $PM_{2.5}$ concentration and an increased risk for viral acute bronchitis [11]. Studies are in progress to examine the effects of indoor particulate matter in children 3–5 years of age [12]. The increased risk for acute viral bronchitis could be due to the damaged airway epithelium resulting from toxic air.

Additionally, there may be additional detrimental effects of poor air quality on the neonate's immature immune system. Air pollution can enhance certain T helper subpopulations and dysregulate anti-viral immune responses [13]. It is well-established that exposure to passive smoking in the family home is a major risk factor for lower respiratory tract (LRT) infection (including bronchitis) for children. A meta-analysis of 60 studies confirmed this risk for those aged 2 years and less [14]. The neonate starts with an immature and therefore impaired immune system and then various early life exposures impact its subsequent immune function [15]. In developing countries factors such as malnutrition, preterm delivery, low birth weight, incomplete immunization and poor feeding practices all contribute to the increased risk for development of acute respiratory tract infection in children [16].

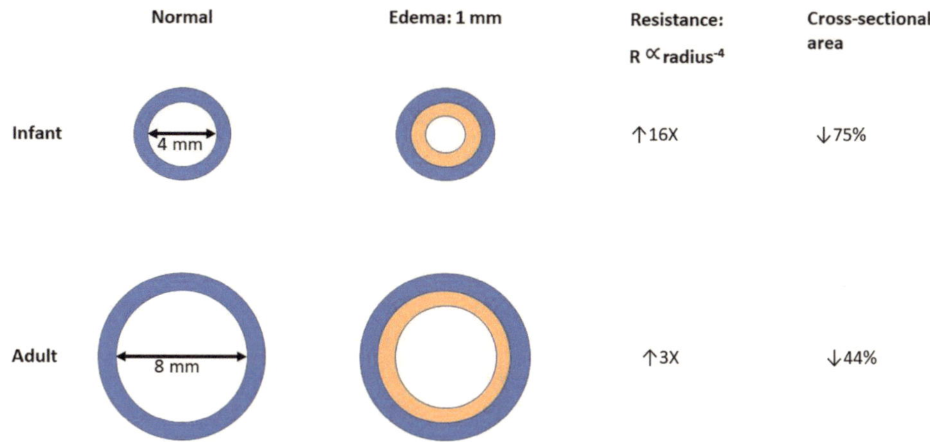

Figure 1.
The effect of airway narrowing in adult and neonate ariways.

Finally, the diameter of the infant's airways is much smaller than that of the adult's. According to Poiseuille's Law, resistance through a cylinder is inversely proportional to its radius to the fourth power (see **Figure 1**). If there is an increase by 1 mm in the bronchial epithelium due to mucus production, edema or swelling from inflammation (whether by viral infection or toxic air inhalation), the airway resistance in an adult airway may increase by three-fold compared with a 16-fold increase in an infant. Therefore, infants and young children will experience much more respiratory difficulty than older children or adults and are more prone to fatigue and subsequent respiratory failure from the increased work in breathing through a narrower airway. Additionally, the 75-fold decrease in cross-sectional area is more pronounced in an infant than in adult (a 44-fold decrease) resulting in an increased propensity to mucus plugs and airway obstruction.

3. Acute bronchitis: etiology

The distinction between infections of the upper respiratory tract (URT) and lower respiratory tracts (LRT) such as bronchitis, bronchiolitis, and pneumonia can be difficult. "Acute bronchitis is a clinical diagnosis characterized by cough due to acute inflammation of the trachea and large airways without evidence of pneumonia. Pneumonia should be suspected in patients with tachypnea, tachycardia, dyspnea, or lung findings suggestive of pneumonia" [17]. In one review of 14 studies conducting in primary care settings, acute cough was mainly caused by URT infections (62%) followed by bronchitis (33%) [18]. Cough associated with acute respiratory tract infections in the ambulatory setting appears to resolve in 50% of children by 10 days and in 90% by 25 days in pooled results from five studies conducted in Western countries [19].

3.1 Viruses

Acute episodes of coughing are usually caused by respiratory viral infections with most commonly identified being rhinovirus, enterovirus, influenza A and B, parainfluenza, coronavirus, human metapneumovirus, and respiratory syncytial virus. Bacteria are detected in 1–10% of cases of acute bronchitis [17]. In contrast it should be noted that the etiology in developing countries is predominantly bacterial [16]. Although respiratory viruses can be the most common cause of acute bronchitis the precise organism is not usually identified because viral cultures and serologic testing are not routinely performed for acute bronchitis in children. However, the recent identification of the severe acute respiratory syndrome coronavirus 2 (SARS-CoV-2) causing coronavirus disease 2019 (COVID-19) has resulted in its rapid detection by home detection kits and confirmation by polymerase chain reaction (PCR)-based laboratory tests. The clinical presentation of COVID-19 can range from asymptomatic, to mild upper respiratory symptoms, acute bronchitis, severe pneumonia and death after multi-organ failure. The most common symptoms of COVID-19 infection in children are cough and fever [20]. Loss of taste or smell are noteworthy and somewhat specific. Other signs and symptoms include cough that becomes productive, chest pain, changes in the skin (such as discoloration areas on the feet or hands, sore throat, nausea with vomiting, abdominal pain or diarrhea; chills, muscle aches and pain, extreme fatigue, new severe headache, and new nasal congestions.

These infections are usually self-limiting and symptoms such as coughing are resolved after a couple weeks. It can be difficult to distinguish between acute viral bronchitis and the common cold or URT infection. "Besides cough, other signs and symptoms of acute bronchitis include sputum production, dyspnea, nasal congestion, headache, and fever...Patients may have substernal or chest wall pain when coughing. Fever is not a typical finding after the first few days...Production of sputum, even purulent, is common and does not correlate with bacterial infection" [17].

3.2 Bacterial and other non-viral infectious causes

Rare bacterial causes such as *Bordetella pertussis, Mycoplasma pneumonia* and *Chlamydophila pneumonia* are important to recognize since specific antibiotics are available and need to be started early to prevent or limit community spread. The presence of posttussive vomiting was found to be moderately sensitive (60%) and specific (66%) in diagnosing pertussis in children. In contrast, for adults both paroxysmal cough and absence of fever had high sensitivity (93.2% and 81.8%, respectively) but low specificity (20.6% and 18.8%). On the other hand, inspiratory whooping and posttussive emesis had low sensitivity (32.5% and 29.8%) but high specificity (77.7% and 79.5%) [21]. The presence of pertussis in over one-third of patients who are still coughing between 2 and 4 weeks [18] is noteworthy in view of evidence that treatment with appropriate antibiotics can limit the spread if given early. Indeed, the BTS guidelines state: "Much coughing in children lasting >3 weeks is related to transient viral or pertussis-like infections" [3]. Surveys of pertussis have emphasized the increased risk of pertussis in adolescents and adults (especially those aged greater than 50 years) in Europe and Asia [22] and in children in Africa [23] (despite high vaccination rates in some areas).

Infection with *Mycoplasma pneumoniae* and *Chlamydophila pneumoniae* are common in children aged 5 years or older [24]. In a review of 7 publications on Mycoplasma pneumonia in children, 91.4% had coughing and 94.2% with fever, but only 23.1% with dyspnea or difficulty breathing and 25.0% were wheezing [25]. The authors concluded their finding is "consistent with other studies that demonstrated no clinical or radiological features to identify Mycoplasma pneumonia."

3.3 Foreign body

The possibility of an inhaled foreign body should always be considered in pediatrics, especially in children less than 3 years of age. Increased tendency for aspiration has been attributed to the child using their mouth to explore their world. They also have immature neuromuscular mechanisms to protect their airway as well as incoordination in swallowing. Additionally, there may be premature efforts by parents or other caretakers to start inappropriate solids or offering high-risk foods (such as peanuts) or having un-supervised mealtimes. Many times the aspiration may not be noticed and a detailed history will not reveal this possibility. A systematic review and meta-analysis of 7 studies specified 6 predictive variables: air trapping, unilateral reduced air entry, witnessed choking, wheezing and suspicious radiographic findings [26]. In a recent single-center study of 726 pediatric patients with confirmed foreign body aspiration coughing was present in 83.9% [27]. Another review of 15 studies (totaling 5606 patients) found no single finding had both positive and negative predictive values over 50%. The "classic triad" (history of an acute event of choking or coughing, wheezing, and unilateral decreased breath sounds) did have 90% specificity but only 35% sensitivity [28]. Obviously, removal of the foreign body will relieve the symptoms and prevent future damage. In some communities flexible bronchoscopy is readily available and should be performed. A review of 23 papers comprising 2588 cases indicated successful removal of the foreign body in 87.1% of cases [29]. When the presence of a foreign body is still uncertain, rigid bronchoscopy or computerized tomography (CT) are other options [30]. Both require general anesthesia and personnel experienced in detection and management of foreign body in young children.

3.4 Environmental factors

Exposure to irritants, odors, allergens, and extreme weather conditions such as cold and/or dry air can also cause acute cough. Not only can poor air quality result in an increased risk for microbial infections, but irritants (both indoors and outdoors) and cigarette smoke can directly affect the airway mucosal surfaces. A review of 7 studies also found adolescent use of e-cigarettes was associated with increased coughing [31]. Peripheral nerve fibers may be activated and mucus glands stimulated to produce mucus. These situations are speculated to result in "neurogenic inflammation of the cough reflex, which becomes hypersensitive," [32] as well as bronchial inflammation with subsequent obstructed airways and stimulation of cough to expectorate the mucus containing the toxic substances and/or allergens. Some make the distinction between "specific acute coughing" which is a response to specific substances and "non-specific." It is the latter which may eventually result in the diagnosis of bronchial asthma.

Childhood asthma can be particularly challenging to detect due to the young age and multiplicity of disease phenotypes. It can present as acute bronchitis or bronchiolitis and resolve as asthma symptoms are usually intermittent. The disease phenotypes are not fixed and may evolve as the child ages until one sees the typical asthma triad of "wheeze, shortness of breath and cough" [33]. Furthermore, their young age makes it difficult to conduct diagnostic tests such as measuring pulmonary function although there have been attempts at obtaining meaningful measurements easily and noninvasively. Other attempts to determine the role of various environmental allergens through *in vitro* or *in vivo* testing are not done at the initial presentation due to their need for subspecialty involvement and relatively invasiveness.

ISPAI [34]	ACCP [1]	ERS [2]
Systemic Redflags		
Neonatal onset of cough		
Digital clubbing	Digital clubbing	Digital clubbing
Failure to thrive	Growth failure	Failure to thrive
Use of medications/drugs		
Palatal abnormalities		
	Feeding difficulties	Feeding difficulties
	Neurodevelopmental abnormality	Neurodevelopmental abnormality
Fever		
	Facial pain/purulent nasal discharge	Recurrent sinopulmonary infections
Pallor		
Sweating		
Dehydration		
Findings suggestive of immunodeficiency		Immunodeficiency
	Recurrent pneumonia	
	Recurrent infections	
		Tuberculosis risk
Pulmonary Redflags		
Chest pain	Chest pain	Chest pain
Daily moist or wet cough	Daily wet/productive cough	
Hemoptysis	Hemoptysis	Haemoptysis
Abnormal cough characteristics		
Tachycardia		
	Cardiac abnormalities	Cardiac abnormalities
Hypoxia/cyanosis	Hypoxia/cyanosis	
	Choked	History suggestive of inhaled foreign body
History of previous lung disease or predisposing causes	Previous history of chronic lung or esophageal disease	
Dyspnea/tachypnea/respiratory distress	Dyspnea or tachypnea	Dyspnea
		Respiratory distress
	Exertional dyspnea	Exertional dyspnaea
Chest shape and chest wall deformities	Chest wall deformity	Chest wall deformity
	Hoarse voice/stridor	
Adventitious lung sounds	Auscultatory findings abnormal	Auscultatory crackles

ISPAI [34]	ACCP [1]	ERS [2]
	Wheeze-monophonic	
	Wheeze-polyphonic	

ISPAC = Italian Society of Pediatric Allergy and Immunology [34]; ACCP = American College of Chest Physicians [1]; and ERS = European Respiratory Society [2].

Table 1.
The use of specific cough pointers by three professional organizations suggesting further evaluation may be needed in children with acute bronchitis.*

In summary, about 90% of cases of acute bronchitis will resolve without any acute intervention after 2 weeks since the main etiology are various respiratory viral infections. However, there may be familial factors such as a family history of asthma or other chronic lung disorders such as cystic fibrosis or bronhiectasis which indicate the need for closer evaluation for other underlying disease processes. Early detection is important since the acute episode may be the first indicating a chronic process. (See discussion on chronic bronchitis in children.) The presence of certain systemic and/or respiratory findings such as failure to thrive or clubbing may result in further evaluation such as chest roentgenogram and/or pulmonary function testing at earlier time periods [2, 3, 34]. These are referred to as "specific cough pointers" and listed in **Table 1**. Any previous episode of choking should prompt consideration for an inhaled foreign body and appropriate referral to a specialist. Finally, one needs to evaluate for any exposure to various environmental factors.

4. Subacute bronchitis

When coughing continues longer than 2 weeks (but less than 8 weeks), it can be labeled as subacute bronchitis. A review of 14 studies conducted mainly in Western countries noted that subacute cough (that is, coughing persisting more than 3 weeks) is caused by recurrent respiratory tract infection (27.7%), asthma (50.4%) and pertussis (37.2%) [18]. The continued presence of viral respiratory infection is consistent with the observation that 10% of children will continue to cough after 25 days [18].

However several mechanisms for a prolonged post-infectious coughing have been postulated: (1) a continued inflammatory process as a result of the immune function to control the infection and (2) irritation caused by drainage of mucus in the nasopharynx or post-nasal drip (PND) [35]. The former can be seen as a similar process in which the inflammatory cells release mediators in response to inhaled allergens in allergic asthma. These mediators can effect nerve fibers, smooth muscles along bronchial airways, endothelial cells lining blood vessels, and/or goblet cells in airway mucus glands. A state of airway hyperreactivity (AHR) may the result of the inflammation, which can become chronic if there is continued exposure to the offending substance.

The BTS had designated the term of "postviral cough" as that cough originally starting with a viral infection of the URT but lasting greater than 3 weeks. "Recurrent cough" represent repeated episodes (at least two times per year) not associated with URT viral infection each one lasting greater than 7–14 days. If there is a clear precipitating trigger (such as exposure to fumes or cigarette smoke) then that cough is a "specific cough." This is to distinguish from "non-specific isolated cough," which typically is described as a persistent dry cough without any other respiratory symptom, no signs of chronic lung disease and a normal chest radiograph [3]. Some in this group may likely represent those with AHR; while others have asthma or cough-variant asthma.

An Australian study described children with a history of wet cough of greater than 3 weeks duration with a significant amount of neutrophils and pathogenic bacteria in their bronchoalveolar fluid (BAL) responding to a two-week treatment with antibiotics (amoxicillin-clavulanate acid) [36]. This condition which they termed protracted bacterial bronchitis (PBB) was redefined by the ERS to exclude the need to obtain BAL by three clinical criteria: "(1) presence of continuous chronic (>4 weeks' duration) wet or productive cough; (2) absence of symptoms or signs (i.e., specific cough pointers) suggestive of other causes of wet or productive cough; and (3) cough resolved following a 2–4 week course of an appropriate oral antibiotic" [2] This definition has been adopted by the ACCP but with a qualifier that children with clinical PBB who also have BAL (or sputum) confirmation of pathogenic bacteria be termed "microbiologically based-PBB (PBB-micro) [1]. The initial description suggested that patients with cough continuing beyond 2 weeks can be further divided into those with a "wet" (69%) or "dry" sounding quality of their cough. Those with the former tend to indicate a specific etiology, the most common which is bacterial infection or PBB (45%) [37]. Other pathogens also included *M. pneumoniae*, *B. pertussis*, and tuberculosis. These findings have been confirmed by numerous investigators with a prevalence varying from 11% to 41% of pulmonary referrals [38]. The most common bacteria include *Haemophilus influenza*e (47–81%) followed by *Streptococcus pneumoniae*, and less commonly *Moraxella catarrhalis* [39]. It appears the presence of *H. influenzae* increases the risk for the development of bronchiectasis [40] as well as recurrent PBB (defined as greater than 3 episodes per year) [31]. PBB and bronchiectasis share many features with chronic suppurative lung disease and some have speculated that these three represent a spectrum of severity with a common underlying pathology with bacterial infection interacting with neutrophilic mediated airway inflammation [41].

5. Management

Although viral respiratory infections account for a majority of acute bronchitis cases, it is important to obtain a detailed clinical history to evaluate the role of various environmental factors such as exposure to tobacco smoke or other irritants (both indoor such as perfumes or wood stove burning and outdoors such as air pollution), allergens from pets, trees, grasses, or weeds, dust, or molds. It is therefore important to evaluate and eliminate these environmental exacerbating factors as much as possible. Also an episode of choking could suggest an inhaled or aspirated foreign body.

Much of the coughing from respiratory viral infections is resolved by 2–3 weeks. There should be some improvement in the second week. Coughing which is relentless and progressive with increased severity (either frequency or severity or both) should prompt further evaluation after 2 weeks. Evaluation for pertussis should be considered sooner when clinical history is suggestive. Specifically, post-tussive vomiting is indicative of pertussis in children. In adolescents and adults the presence of whooping or post-tussive vomiting should rule in a possible diagnosis of pertussis and absence of paroxysmal cough or presence of fever should rule it out. Detection by PCR appears to be the most useful. Appropriate antibiotics (that is, macrolide) are given for prophylaxis of household contacts or those exposed who are at high risk of severe illness (such as infants, immunocompromised individuals) but they do not shorten the duration of coughing or hospitalization rate [42]. Azithromycin and clarithromycin appear to be equally effective but the former may have less side effects and is given once a day for 5 days. If given very early (in the first 1–2 weeks) it the disease, it can slightly alter the clinical course but their main role is to reduce the period of infectivity. However since the early stages of pertussis can be difficult to distinguish from a simple head cold, this recommendation is difficult to carry out in practice other than in the situation when coughing starts after a known exposure" [3]. A Cochrane review did not indicate any effective treatment for pertussis cough [43] and the duration can be quite prolonged. The median duration in unimmunized children less than 6 years was 52 to 61 days 29 to 39 days for those who received the pertussis vaccine [44].

As mentioned earlier, the possibility of infection with other atypical bacteria such as *Mycoplasma pneumonia* and *Chlamydia* should also be considered with prolonged coughing. Screening for tuberculosis should be done in high risk patient populations as well as in areas where TB is prevalent. Establishing the presence of *Mycoplasma* or *Chlamydia* is more difficult since serological tests alone do not distinguish Mycoplasma infection from carriage [45]. It appears that detection by PCR can be useful [46]. Antibiotic treatment for these two organisms is controversial. A Cochrane review of 7 studies involving 1912 children concluded there was insufficient evidence to make any specific recommendations due to lack of high quality (double blinded, placebo controlled) studies although one controlled study indicated 100% of children treated with azithromycin had clinical resolution compared to 77% untreated children after 1 month of follow-up [47].

It is always difficult to decide whether the episode of acute bronchitis represent the first attack of bronchial asthma. Pulmonary function testing can be performed to detect those children with asthma. Spirometry is often available and can be reliably used in children aged greater than 6 years and in some younger if trained pediatric personnel are conducting the tests [1]. However, ACCP does note that neither spirometry nor CXR are sensitive (i.e., normal results do not imply absence of disease) but they are specific (i.e., abnormal results do indicate presence of some respiratory illness). However, a systematic review of the use of spirometry did not find any randomized controlled trials demonstrating its use in improved clinical outcomes in children [48]. Part of the problem is that tests showing AHR are sensitive but not specific for asthma. Children may develop temporary AHR and an asthma-like transient clinical syndrome due to post-infectious processes (such as following infections with respiratory syncytial virus or *M pneumonia*) and in association with upper respiratory allergies such as allergic rhinitis. There is no relation to the child's post-infectious AHR and subsequent development of asthma or response to asthma medications (such as inhaled albuterol or salbutamol and inhaled corticosteroids). There is difficulty in making a firm diagnosis of asthma because while "almost all children with asthma have intermittent cough, wheeze and/or exercise-induced symptoms, only about a quarter of children with these symptoms have asthma" as cited by ACCP [1]. Another variable is the type of challenge used to measure AHR with some suggesting exercise-stress testing over methacholine inhalation as being more sensitive for asthma. Therefore, those children who have isolated chronic cough and no wheezing should be followed and monitored closely. A 10-year follow-up suggest up to 45% do develop asthma and AHR (by methacholine challenge) is a strong risk factor [49]. Some have labeled them as "cough-variant asthma" but others believe that this is a misnomer and represent a problem of over-diagnosis of asthma. The ERS does recognize three subgroups of asthmatic cough with classic asthma characterized by airflow variability and AHR and diagnosed with improvement in spirometry variables after bronchodilators. Cough variant asthma have cough as the sole symptom and is improved with bronchodilators. The third form is eosinophilic bronchitis [2].

Unfortunately examination for the presence of eosinophilia in the blood, BAL fluid, sputum or bronchial biopsy (which is helpful in diagnosing adult asthma) is not rewarding in children and is quite invasive or difficult to obtain. Although there is strong evidence that measurement of fractional exhaled nitric oxide (F_{eNO}) may indicate eosinophilic involvement in the lungs, there have been conflicting results on its utility in evaluating cough in children [2]. Part of the problem are the presence of variability among detection methods and the different and varied patient populations being studied. Therefore, both the ACCP and ERS concluded that there is no good study using F_{eNO} levels as a reliable diagnostic indicator for asthma and also as predictor for anti-inflammatory response in treatment [1, 2].

5.1 Treatment

Management of acute bronchitis mainly consists of supportive care and possibly treatment of the more bothersome symptoms. Most guidelines stress the "trivial and self-limiting problem" of acute cough but recognize it does result in the child's discomfort and can cause in loss of sleep for entire family [35]. The problem is a general lack of good studies showing both efficacy and safety of currently available medications, both over-the-counter and prescription. Therefore, there is a "wait-and-see" strategy for acute bronchitis [18], especially if it occurs during the winter-time when there is high prevalence of viral URTI in the community and in otherwise healthy children.

5.2 Medications

A recent systemic review of 34 studies on the use of non-steroidal anti-inflammatory drugs (NSAIDs) in acute viral respiratory tract infections showed these medications were beneficial in relieving fever and sore throat but not cough [50]. Another review by Cochrane of 30 studies (children included in 9) on the use of antihistamine-decongestant-analgesic combinations indicate "no evidence of effectiveness in young children" but "some general benefits in adults and older children" [51].

Two recent randomized controlled pediatric trials with local herbal remedies such as a root extract from *Pelargonium sidoides* in Africa [52] and Jiuwei Zhuhuang powder consisting of nine herbs in China [53] indicated their use significantly decreased the cough frequency over placebo in the first study or decreased the cough duration by 1 day over an antihistamine (chlorphenamine)-decongestant (cowbenzor)-analgesic (paracetamol) in the second study. These studies represent a growing interest to use natural remedies for acute viral respiratory infections in view of their apparent safety and the current lack of any effective cough relievers [54]. A Cochrane review of honey concluded "honey probably relieves cough symptoms to a greater extent than no treatment, diphenhydramine, and placebo; but may make little or no difference compared to dextromethorphan. Honey probably reduces cough duration better than placebo and salbutamol. There was no strong evidence for or against using honey" [55].

Although dextromethorphan (which is a non-opioid synthetic derivative of morphine) has been shown in three placebo-controlled trials to decrease cough frequency when compared with placebo [56] there are potential side-effects and safety concerns regarding its use in pediatrics. At higher doses there are psychoactive effects and therefore a potential for abuse [57]. A review of hydrocodone/chorpheniramine also did not reveal any "robust efficacy data" in the relief of cough and respiratory symptoms associated with allergy or viral URIs in pediatrics [58]. Therefore, previous ACCP guidelines emphasized the lack of efficacy and potential morbidity and mortality of over-the-counter (OTC) cough medications in young children for cough [59]. Subsequently, the United States Federal Drug Administration (FDA) issued a warning and encouraged manufacturers to re-labeled these products "do not use in children under 4 years of age." Later the FDA also limited prescription opioid cough and cold medications to those greater than 18 years of age.

The updated ACCP guidelines [1] state "other than honey...OTC cough medications have little, if any, benefit in the symptomatic control of acute cough in children but importantly, preparations containing anti-histamine and dextromethorphan were associated with adverse events. Thus, using OTC medications has to be balanced with [potential] adverse events...For children with acute cough, we suggest that the use of over the counter cough and cold medicines should not be prescribed until they have been shown to make cough less severe or resolve sooner...honey may offer more relief for cough symptoms than no treatment, diphenhydramine, or placebo, but it is not better than dextromethorphan...suggest avoiding codeine-containing medications because of the potential for serious side effects." A recent Cochrane review indicated some general benefit in adults and older children with antihistamine-analgesic-decongestant combinations for the common cold but "these benefits must be weighed against the risk of adverse effects. There is no evidence of effectiveness in young children" [51].

The rationale behind the use of antihistamines is the possible role of allergy in acute bronchitis. The presence of mucus in the bronchial tubes may be difficult to expel due to the narrowed airway and the inadequacy of the cough reflex. Additionally, there may be production of mucus in the nasopharynx which descends through the pharynx causing persistent mechanical stimulation of the upper portion of the larynx [35]. The process could be triggered from atopic or allergic factors as well concomitant infection causing acute as well as chronic inflammation of the upper airways. Because of the multiple etiologies which can include not only various rhinitis and sinusitis phenotypes but also various anatomic abnormalities, chemical-induced rhinitis, etc., "a uniform definition of upper airway cough syndrome (UACS) with post-nasal drip (PND) is lacking across the United States, Europe, and Asia" [60]. Diagnosis is mainly clinical since radiographic studies such as conventional sinus radiograph or paranasal Water view or paranasal sinus CT are limited with low sensitivity and low specificity. Therefore, the ACCP, American Academy of Pediatrics, Infectious Diseases Society of America all do not recommend routine radiological assessment. Unfortunately there are no randomized control trials on therapies for UACS examining the effect on cough. One study on allergic rhinitis did find a significant decrease nasal symptoms and daytime cough (but not nighttime cough) using topical corticosteroids (mometasone furoate) [61]. If sinusitis is suspected, the recommended first-line therapy is antibiotics (amoxicillin or amoxicillin-clavulanate) for 7–10 days for acute (>10 days) and 20 days for chronic (>90 days) sinusitis [2].

There is no role for antibiotics in acute bronchitis (without concomitant sinusitis) since the etiology is not bacterial. However, there continues to be a tendency for physicians to prescribe amoxicillin, amoxicillin-clavulanate or azithromycin in almost 40% cases of acute bronchitis, laryngitis, and rhinopharyngitis [62]. It is difficult to determine whether they were seriously considering the possibility of pertussis or the atypical bacteria (i.e., *Mycoplasma* or *Chlamycia*) as mentioned above. Additionally, in contrast to the usual dry cough from infection by atypical bacteria, a wet cough may develop and persist for greater than 3 weeks raising the possibility of protracted bacterial bronchitis (PBB) [37]. Since part of the definition is the child's response to 2–4 weeks of antibiotics the practitioner needs to critically evaluate and decide whether an empiric trial of antibiotics is needed after 2 weeks of coughing. ACCP guidelines do recommend that "children aged ≤ 14 years chronic (>4 weeks duration) wet or productive cough unrelated to an underlying disease and without any other specific cough pointers 2 weeks of antibiotics targeted to common respiratory bacteria (Streptococcus pneumonia, *Haemophilus influenza, Moraxella catarrhalis*) targeted to local antibiotic sensitivities" [1]. If there is a response within 2 weeks, then the diagnosis of PBB can be made. If there is no response after 2 weeks, an additional 2 weeks of antibiotic(s) should be done A recent randomized controlled trial indicated that an initial 4-week antibiotic course in suspected PBB led to a longer cough-free period than a 2 week duration [63]. ERS also agreed that a "trial of antibiotics is suggested in children with chronic wet cough with normal chest radiographs, normal spirometry and no warning signs" [2]. If there is no response after a total of 4 weeks of antibiotics, then further investigations such as flexible bronchoscopy with cultures and/or chest computerized tomography (CT) should be considered as further diagnostic procedures since the condition has now evolved into chronic bronchitis with coughing duration of greater than 4 weeks.

If a trial of asthma therapy is warranted in selected patients (see above discussion on Management), inhaled corticosteroids (ICS) are suggested. The ACCP recommends 400 mcg/day equivalent of budesonide or beclomethasone "as this dose is effective in the management of most childhood asthma and adverse events occur on higher doses" and reassess in 2 to 4 weeks. However, if there is a response, the child "does not necessarily have asthma and the child should be re-evaluated off asthma treatment as resolution of cough may occur with the period effect (spontaneous resolution or a transient effect responsive to ICS use" [1]. This is due to a Cochrane review that indicate no benefit from ICS in treatment with non-specific chronic cough related to asthma [64]. The ERS suggests that ICS may be less effective "since inflammation in cough-variant asthma and eosinophilic bronchitis is located in different parts of the airway from that seen in classic asthma, and may be drive by other pathways such as the innate immune system" [2]. Indeed, inhalation of bronchodilators (alone) or anticholinergics are not effective for the non-specific or asthmatic-like cough. Therefore, a trial of systemic anti-leukotriene medication was suggested for adults but the relatively high incidence (>10%) of mild and transient neuropsychiatric adverse side-effect preclude their empiric use in children. ACCP guidelines did mention older studies showing resolution of cough after 2 weeks of oral theophylline or inhaled mast cell stabilizers (cromoglycate or nedocromil). There was no mention of the role for combined low-dose ICS and long-acting beta 2 agonist but ERS noted a lack of any good studies examining their use in cough-variant asthma and asthmatic cough.

6. Conclusions

Acute and chronic bronchitis represent a spectrum of disease involving the lower airways. The most common etiology is a respiratory viral infection which usually causes short-lived coughing lasting less than 2–3 weeks in 90% of cases and resolves without any complications. The cough results from viral infection of epithelial cells and shedding of necrotic cells into the airway exposing sensory nerve endings. Attempts to control the infection involve the production of cytokines causing vascular leak, mucus secretion, and recruitment of inflammatory cells. These result in some blockage of the airway which may further invoke coughing to remove the mixture of secretions and mucus. Coughing resolves with control of the viral infection.

Some children may require a longer time to heal with bronchial epithelium regeneration and down-regulating the immune response. The injured epithelial surface may be at increased risk for bacterial superinfection, which will then require the use of antimicrobial medications. This process may be similar to viral infections of the upper airways producing croup which may then progress to bacterial tracheitis. Other children may have an initial infection with nonviral pathogens which will persist and result in prolonged coughing. Involvement of tuberculosis, mycoplasma and chlamydia has to be evaluated taking into account the surrounding community. Environmental factors such as exposure to cigarette smoke, perfumes, etc., need to be examined and managed accordingly. The possibility of an inhaled foreign body should always be considered.

Author details

Terry Chin
Department of Pediatric Pulmonary/Allergy and Immunology, Miller Children's Hospital, Long Beach, University of California, Irvine, CA, USA

*Address all correspondence to: twchin1224@gmail.com

References

[1] Chang AB, Oppenheimer JJ, Irwin RS, CHEST Expert Cough Panel. Managing chronic cough as a symptom in children and management algorithms: CHEST Guideline and Expert Panel Report. Chest. 2020;**158**(1):303-329

[2] Morice AH, Millqvist E, Bieksiene K, et al. ERS guidelines on the diagnosis and treatment of chronic cough in adults and children. The European Respiratory Journal. 2020;**55**:1901136. DOI: 10.1183/13993003.01136-2019

[3] Shields MD, Bush A, Everard ML, McKenzie S, Primhak R, British Thoracic Society Cough Guideline Group. BTS guidelines: Recommendations for the assessment and management of cough in children. Thorax. 2008;**63**(Suppl. 3):iii1-iii5. DOI: 10.1136/thx.2007.077370

[4] Lai K, Shen H, Zhou X, Qiu Z, Cai S, Huang K, et al. Clinical practice guidelines for diagnosis and Management of Cough-Chinese Thoracic Society (CTS) asthma consortium. Journal of Thoracic Disease. 2018;**10**(11):6314-6351

[5] Kohno S, Ishida T, Uchida Y, et al. The Japanese Respiratory Society guidelines for management of cough. Respirology. 2006;**11**(Suppl. 4):S135-S136

[6] Liang H, Ye W, Wang Z, et al. Prevalence of chronic cough in China: A systematic review and meta-analysis. BMC Pulmonary Medicine. 2022;**22**:62. DOI: 10.1186/s12890-022-01847-w

[7] Irwin RS, French CL, Chang AB, Altman KW, CHEST Expert Cough Panel. Classification of cough as a symptom in adults and management algorithms: CHEST Guideline and Expert Panel Report. Chest. 2018;**153**(1):196-209. DOI: 10.1016/j.chest.2017.10.016

[8] Di Cicco M, Kantar A, Masini B, Nuzzi G, Ragazzo V, Peroni D. Structural and functional development in airways throughout childhood: Children are not small adults. Pediatric Pulmonology. 2021;**56**(1):240-251. DOI: 10.1002/ppul.25169

[9] Schwartz J. Air pollution and children's health. Pediatrics. 2004;**113**(4 Suppl):1037-1043

[10] Ziou M, Tham R, Wheeler AJ, Graeme R, Stephens N, Johnston FH. Outdoor particulate matter exposure and upper respiratory tract infections in children and adolescents: A systematic review and meta-analysis. Environmental Research. 2022;**210**:112969. DOI: 10.1016/j.envres.2022.112969

[11] Chen PC, Mou CH, Chen CW, Hsieh DPH, Tsai SP, Wei CC, et al. Roles of ambient temperature and $PM_{2.5}$ on childhood acute bronchitis and bronchiolitis from viral infection. Viruses. 2022;**14**(9):1932. DOI: 10.3390/v14091932

[12] Thornburg J, Halchenko Y, McCombs M, Siripanichgon N, Dowell E, Cho SH, et al. Children's particulate matter exposure characterization as part of the New Hampshire Birth Cohort Study. International Journal of Environmental Research and Public Health. 2021;**18**(22):12109. DOI: 10.3390/ijerph182212109

[13] Glencross DA, Ho T-R, Camina N, Hawrylowicz CM, Pfeffer PE. Air pollution and its effects on the immune system. Free Radical Biology and Medicine. 2020;**151**:56-68. DOI: 10.1016/j.freeradbiomed.2020.01.179

[14] Jones LL, Hashim A, McKeever T, Cook DG, Britton J, Leonardi-Bee J. Parental and household smoking and the

increased risk of bronchitis, bronchiolitis and other lower respiratory infections in infancy: Systematic review and meta-analysis. Respiratory Research. 2011;**12**(1):5. DOI: 10.1186/1465-9921-12-5

[15] Bermick J, Schaller M. Epigenetic regulation of pediatric and neonatal immune responses. Pediatric Research. 2022;**91**:297-327. DOI: 10.1038/s41390-021-01630-3

[16] Shah S, Malde T, Nayakpara D. Risk factors associated with acute respiratory infection in children among one month to 5 years. International Journal of Pediatrics and Geriatrics. 2022;**5**(1):6-10. DOI: 10.33545/26643685.2022.v5.i1a.151

[17] Kinkade S, Long NA. Acute bronchitis. American Family Physician. 2016;**94**(7):560-565

[18] Bergmann M, Haasenritter J, Beidatsch D, Schwarm S, Hörner K, Bösner S, et al. Coughing children in family practice and primary care: A systematic review of prevalence, etiology and prognosis. BMC Pediatrics. 2021;**21**(1):260. DOI: 10.1186/s12887-021-02739-4

[19] Thompson M, Vodicka TA, Blair PS, Buckley DI, Heneghan C, Hay AD, et al. Duration of symptoms of respiratory tract infections in children: Systematic review. British Medical Journal. 2013;**347**:f7027. DOI: 10.1136/bmj.f7027

[20] Mayo Clinic. Coronavirus in babies and children. December 17, 2022. Available at: https://www.mayoclinic.org/diseases-conditions/coronavirus/in-depth/coronavirus-in-babies-and-children/art-20484405 [Accessed: March 01, 2023]

[21] Moore A, Harnden A, Grant CC, Patel S, Irwin RS, CHEST Expert Cough Panel. Clinically diagnosing pertussis-associated cough in adults and children: CHEST Guideline and Expert Panel Report. Chest. 2019;**155**(1):147-154. DOI: 10.1016/j.chest.2018.09.027

[22] Macina D, Evans KE. Bordetella pertussis in school-age children, adolescents and adults: A systematic review of epidemiology and mortality in Europe. Infectious Disease and Therapy. 2021;**10**(4):2071-2118. DOI: 10.1007/s40121-021-00520-9

[23] Macina D, Evans KE. Bordetella pertussis in school-age children, adolescents, and adults: A systematic review of epidemiology, burden, and mortality in Africa. Infectious Disease and Therapy. 2021;**10**(3):1097-1113. DOI: 10.1007/s40121-021-00442-6

[24] Leung AKC, Wong AHC, Hon KL. Community-acquired pneumonia in children. Recent Patient in Inflammatory Allergy Drug Discovery. 2018;**12**(2):136-144. DOI: 10.2174/1872213X12666180621163821

[25] Kevat PM, Morpeth M, Graham H, Gray AZ. A systematic review of the clinical features of pneumonia in children aged 5-9 years: Implications for guidelines and research. Journal of Global Health. 2022;**12**:10002. DOI: 10.7189/jogh.12.10002

[26] Lee JJW, Philteos J, Levin M, Namavarian A, Propst EJ, Wolter NE. Clinical prediction models for suspected pediatric foreign body aspiration: A systematic review and meta-analysis. JAMA Otolaryngology. Head & Neck Surgery. 2021;**147**(9):787-796. DOI: 10.1001/jamaoto.2021.1548

[27] Ulas AB, Aydin Y, Eroglu A. Foreign body aspirations in children and adults. American Journal of Surgery. 2022;**224**(4):1168-1173. Available online May 27, 2022. DOI: 10.1016/j.amjsurg.2022.05.032

[28] Zoizner-Agar G, Merchant S, Wang B, April MM. Yield of preoperative findings in pediatric airway foreign bodies—A meta-analysis. International Journal of Pediatric Otorhinolaryngology. 2020;**139**:110442. DOI: 10.1016/j.ijporl.2020.110442

[29] Chantzaras AP, Panagiotou P, Karageorgos S, Douros K. A systematic review of using flexible bronchoscopy to remove foreign bodies from pediatric patients. Acta Paediatrica. 2022;**111**(7):1301-1312. DOI: 10.1111/apa.16351

[30] Gibbons AT, Casar Berazaluce AM, Hanke RE, McNinch NL, Person A, Mehlman T, et al. Avoiding unnecessary bronchoscopy in children with suspected foreign body aspiration using computed tomography. Journal of Pediatric Surgery. 2020;**55**(1):176-181. DOI: 10.1016/j.jpedsurg.2019.09.045

[31] Bourke M, Sharif N, Narayan O. Association between electronic cigarette use in children and adolescents and coughing a systematic review. Pediatric Pulmonology. 2021;**56**(10):3402-3409. DOI: 10.1002/ppul.25619

[32] Rouadi PW, Idriss SA, Bousquet J, Laidlaw TM, Azar CR, et al. WAO-ARIA consensus on chronic cough—Part 1: Role of TRP channels in neurogenic inflammation of cough neuronal pathways. World Allergy Organization Journal. 2021;**14**(12):100617. DOI: 10.1016/j.waojou.2021.100617

[33] Martin J, Townshend J, Brodlie M. Diagnosis and management of asthma in children. BMJ Paediatric Open. 2022;**6**(1):e001277. DOI: 10.1136/bmjpo-2021-001277

[34] Marseglia GL, Manti S, Chiappini E, Brambilla I, Caffarelli C, Calvani M, et al. Acute cough in children and adolescents: A systematic review and a practical algorithm by the Italian Society of Pediatric Allergy and Immunology. Allergological Immunopathology (Madras). 2021;**49**(2):155-169. DOI: 10.15586/aei.v49i2.45

[35] Murgia V, Manti S, Licari A, De Filippo M, Ciprandi G, Marseglia GL. Upper respiratory tract infection-associated acute cough and the urge to cough: New insights for clinical practice. Pediatric Allergy, Immunology and Pulmonology. 2020;**33**(1):3-11. DOI: 10.1089/ped.2019.1135

[36] Marchant JM, Brent MI, Taylor SM, Cox NC, Seymour GJ, Chang AB. Evaluation and outcome of young children with chronic cough. Chest. 2006;**129**:1132-1141. DOI: 10.1378/chest.129.5.1132

[37] Marchant JM, Masters IB, Taylor SM, Chang AB. Utility of signs and symptoms of chronic cough in predicting specific cause in children. Thorax. 2006;**61**:694-698. DOI: 10.1136/thx.2005.056986

[38] Gallucci M, Pedretti M, Giannetti A, di Palmo E, Bertelli L, Pession A, et al. When the cough does not improve: A review on protracted bacterial bronchitis in children. Frontiers in Pediatrics. 2020;**8**:433. DOI: 10.3389/fped.2020.00433

[39] Di Filippo P, Scaparrotta A, Petrosino MI, Attanasi M, Di Pillo S, Chiarelli F, et al. An underestimated cause of chronic cough: The protracted bacterial bronchitis. Annals of Thoracic Medicine. 2018;**13**:7-13

[40] Ruffles TJC, Marchant JM, Masters IB, Yerkovich ST, Wurzel DF, Gibson PG, et al. Outcomes of protracted bacterial bronchitis in children: A 5-year prospective cohort study. Respirology.

2021;**26**(3):241-248. DOI: 10.1111/resp.13950

[41] Chang AB, Redding GJ, Everard ML. Chronic wet cough: Protracted bronchitis, chronic suppurative lung disease and bronchiectasis. Pediatric Pulmonology. 2008;**43**:519-531. DOI: 10.1002/ppul.20821

[42] Kline JM, Smith EA, Zavala A. Pertussis: Common questions and answers. American Family Physician. 2021;**104**(2):186-192

[43] Wang K, Bettiol S, Thompson MJ, Roberts NW, Perera R, Heneghan CJ, et al. Symptomatic treatment of the cough in whooping cough. Cochrane Database of Systematic Reviews. 2014;**2014**(9):CD003257. DOI: 10.1002/14651858.CD003257.pub5

[44] Tozzi AE, Rava L, Ciofidegli Atti ML, et al. Clinical presentation of pertussis in unvaccinated and vaccinated children in the first six years of life. Pediatrics. 2003;**112**(5):1069-1075

[45] Meyer Sauteur PM, Unger WW, Nadal D, Berger C, Vink C, van Rossum AM. Infection with and carriage of mycoplasma pneumoniae in children. Frontiers in Microbiology. 2016;7:329. DOI: 10.3389/fmicb.2016.00329

[46] Rueda ZV, Aguilar Y, Maya MA, López L, Restrepo A, Garcés C, et al. Etiology and the challenge of diagnostic testing of community-acquired pneumonia in children and adolescents. BMC Pediatrics. 2022;**22**(1):169. DOI: 10.1186/s12887-022-03235-z

[47] Gardiner SJ, Gavranich JB, Chang AB. Antibiotics for community-acquired lower respiratory tract infections secondary to Mycoplasma pneumoniae in children. Cochrane Database of Systematic Reviews. 2015;**1**:CD004875. DOI: 10.1002/14651858.CD004875.pub5

[48] Boonjindasup W, Chang AB, McElrea MS, Yerkovich ST, Marchant JM. Does the routine use of spirometry improve clinical outcomes in children?-A systematic review. Pediatric Pulmonology. 2022;**57**(10):2390-2397. DOI: 10.1002/ppul.26045

[49] Nishimura H, Mochizuki H, Tokuyama K, Morikawa A. Relationship between bronchial hyperresponsiveness and development of asthma in children with chronic cough. Pediatric Pulmonology. 2001;**31**(6):415-418. DOI: 10.1002/ppul.1068

[50] Azh N, Barzkar F, Motamed-Gorji N, Pourvali-Talatappeh P, Moradi Y, Vesal Azad R, et al. Nonsteroidal anti-inflammatory drugs in acute viral respiratory tract infections: An updated systematic review. Pharmacology Research & Perspectives. 2022;**10**(2):e00925. DOI: 10.1002/prp2.925

[51] De Sutter AI, Eriksson L, van Driel ML. Oral antihistamine-decongestant-analgesic combinations for the common cold. Cochrane Database of Systematic Reviews. 2022;**1**(1):CD004976. DOI: 10.1002/14651858.CD004976.pub4

[52] Gökçe Ş, Dörtkardeşler BE, Yurtseven A, Kurugöl Z. Effectiveness of Pelargonium sidoides in pediatric patients diagnosed with uncomplicated upper respiratory tract infection: A single-blind, randomized, placebo-controlled study. European Journal of Pediatrics. 2021;**180**(9):3019-3028. DOI: 10.1007/s00431-021-04211-y

[53] Luo H, Song GH, Ma XJ, Sun MM, Zhang M, Xie JR, et al. Effect of Jiuwei

Zhuhuang powder on cough resolution in children with upper respiratory tract infections: A Multicenter Randomized Controlled Trial. Chinese Journal of Integrative Medicine. 2022;**28**(5):387-393. DOI: 10.1007/s11655-021-3462-x

[54] Murgia V, Ciprandi G, Votto M, De Filippo M, Tosca MA, Marseglia GL. Natural remedies for acute post-viral cough in children. Allergological Immunopathological (Madras). 2022;**49**(3):173-184. DOI: 10.15586/aei.v49i3.71

[55] Oduwole O, Udoh EE, Oyo-Ita A, Meremikwu MM. Honey for acute cough in children. Cochrane Database of Systematic Reviews. 2018;**4**(4):CD007094. DOI: 10.1002/14651858.CD007094.pub5

[56] Smith SM, Schroeder K, Fahey T. Over-the-counter (OTC) medications for acute cough in children and adults in community settings. Cochrane Database of Systematic Reviews. 2014;**11**:CD001831. DOI: 10.1002/14651858.CD001831.pub5

[57] Green JL, Wang GS, Reynolds KM, Banner W, Bond GR, Kauffman RE, et al. Safety profile of cough and cold medication use in pediatrics. Pediatrics. 2017;**139**(6):e20163070. DOI: 10.1542/peds.2016-3070

[58] Sloan VS, Jones A, Maduka C, Bentz JWG. A benefit risk review of pediatric use of hydrocodone/chlorpheniramine, a prescription opioid antitussive agent for the treatment of cough. Real World Outcomes. 2019;**6**(2):47-57. DOI: 10.1007/s40801-019-0152-6

[59] Chang AB, Glomb WB. Guidelines for evaluating chronic cough in pediatrics: ACCP evidence based clinical practice guidelines. Chest. 2006;**129**(suppl. 1):260S-283S

[60] Rouadi PW, Idriss SA, Bousquet J, Laidlaw TM, Azar CR, Al-Ahmad MS, et al. WAO-ARIA consensus on chronic cough—Part III: Management strategies in primary and cough-specialty care. Updates in COVID-19. World Allergy Organization Journal. 2022;**15**(5):100649. DOI: 10.1016/j.waojou.2021.10061862

[61] Gawchik S, Goldstein S, Prenner B, et al. Relief of cough and nasal symptoms associated with allergic rhinitis by mometaone furoate nasal spray. Annals of Allergy, Asthma & Immunology. 2003;**90**(4):416-421

[62] Umarovich RO, Rashidovich NR. Antibacterial therapy in the treatment of acute and chronic bronchitis. SCHOLASTIC: Journal of Natural and Medical Education. 2023;**2**(1):101-103

[63] Ruffles TJC, Goyal V, Marchant JM, Masters IB, Yerkovich S, Buntain H, et al. Duration of amoxicillin-clavulanate for protracted bacterial bronchitis in children (DACS): A multi-centre, double blind, randomized controlled trial. The Lancet Respiratory Medicine. 2021;**9**(10):1121-1129. DOI: 10.1016/S2213-2600(21)00104-1

[64] Tomerak AA, McGlashan B, Vyas HH, McKean MC. Inhaled corticosteroids for non-specific chronic cough in children. Cochrane Database of Systematic Reviews. 2005;**4**:CD004231

Chapter 3

Kinesitherapy and Ultrahigh-Frequency Current in Children with Bronchial Asthma

Vyara Dimitrova, Assen Aleksiev and Penka Perenovska

Abstract

The aim is to compare the effect of the combination of kinesitherapy and ultrahigh-frequency current in children with bronchial asthma with a control group without rehabilitation. There were 24 children with bronchial asthma of average age of 8 followed for 10 days. They were randomized into two groups—12 children in the "physiotherapeutic" and 12 in the "control." All were treated with equal standard pharmacotherapy. The first group was treated also with kinesitherapy and ultrahigh-frequency current. At the beginning and end of the therapeutic course, the spirometric and anthropometric parameters were documented. In the statistical analysis were included the proportions between the actual and the expected spirometric parameters, adjusted for all anthropometric parameters. The ratios between the actual and the expected spirometric parameters improved significantly in both groups after 10-day treatment compared with before treatment ($P < 0.05$). In the "physiotherapeutic" group, the improvement after the treatment was significantly greater, when compared with the "control" group ($P < 0.05$). In conclusion, there is a significant therapeutic effect, upgrading that of pharmacotherapy when children with bronchial asthma were treated for 10 days with the combination of kinesitherapy and ultrahigh-frequency current.

Keywords: bronchial asthma, pediatrics, rehabilitation, physiotherapy, kinesitherapy

1. Introduction

Bronchial asthma affects about 300 million people worldwide according to the Global Initiative for Asthma (GINA) [1]. It is a serious global health problem that influences all age groups. The cost of treating these patients is increasing, especially if there is an overlying infection—pneumonia or bronchiectasis disease, as well as its social significance in the community and family [2], manifesting in the young age group. The problem is exacerbated in developing countries, in low-status families where asthma patients are exposed to harmful influences such as cigarette smoke, mold, cockroaches, and other allergens.

According to the National Heart, Lung, and Blood Institute (NHLBI) [3], of the 25 million asthma patients in the USA, 5% (1.25 million) suffer from severe asthma. Asthma is also the most common chronic disease in childhood, affecting over 7% of children [4–8]. About 500,000 people suffer from asthma In Bulgaria, 15,000 are children [4, 6–8]. About 80% of the people with bronchial asthma are diagnosed before their 6th year, and boys, in a ratio of 1:4, are more often affected than girls [7, 8].

Kinesitherapy is used in children with bronchial asthma due to its ability to counteract the consequences on the musculoskeletal system that negatively affect the respiratory system: respiratory muscle imbalance—expiratory muscles (rectus abdominis muscle, abdominal oblique muscles, internal intercostal muscles) are lengthened with decreased tone and strength, while inspiratory muscles (scalene muscles, external intercostal muscles, upper part of trapezius muscle, levator scapulae muscle) are shortened with increased tone and spasm, increased cervical lordosis, increased anterior-posterior chest size, increased thoracic kyphosis, lower rib descent, "gothic shoulders," "barrel-shaped" chest, "shortened" neck, reduced diaphragmatic breathing, raised and forward shoulder girdle, reduced chest mobility, reduced lung volumes and capacities [1, 9–12]. These changes are preventable with adequate kinesitherapy [10, 13]. Some authors think that excessive exercise may provoke an attack, and that is a consideration against kinesitherapy in children with asthma [14, 15]. But the consequences of lack of exercise are detraining, easier fatigue, reduced tolerance to daily exertion, obesity, lethargy, and increased stress [1, 10, 13–15]. By warming up exercises, asthma attacks can be controlled [10, 13–15]. Exercise training can reduce the frequency and severity of asthma attacks induced by excessive physical exercise [1, 10, 13–15]. In addition, increased and more rapid muscle contractions and co-contractions as a consequence of exercises have a broncho-dilating effect [1, 9–15].

Regarding the combination of ultrahigh-frequency current (UHF) and kinesitherapy, there are no studies on asthma in children, despite their hypothetical synergistic broncho-dilating effect. In adult patients with bronchial UHF, an anti-inflammatory and broncho-dilating effect was found, thanks to the endogenous heat effect, which does not burden the thermoregulatory, respiratory, and cardiovascular systems [5, 9, 11, 12]. The reason is that the skin is not a barrier to UHF, and endogenous heat is generated indirectly in depth by the transformation of electromagnetic external energy into kinetic energy of tissue dipoles [5, 9, 11, 12]. This results in tissue heating by the high-frequency oscillations of the dipoles, attempting to head with their positive and negative poles to the high-frequency reversal of the external electromagnetic polarity [5, 9, 11, 12]. Furthermore, endogenous heat from UHF is selective—it can thermally burden tissues with high or low water content, depending on the type of electrodes [5, 9, 11, 12].

The comparison of the effect of the combination of kinesitherapy and ultrahigh-frequency current in children with bronchial asthma versus a control group without rehabilitation is the aim of the work.

2. Material and methods

In the Children's Clinic of the "Alexandrovska" University Hospital (CCAUH), there were 24 children with bronchial asthma of average age of 8 followed for 10 days. They were randomized into two groups—12 children in the "physiotherapeutic" group and 12 children in the "control" group. All children were treated with the same standard pharmacotherapy [1]. In the treatment of the first group ("physiotherapeutic") kinesitherapy and ultrahigh-frequency current were also added.

The algorithm used in the ultrahigh-frequency current treatment was as follows: the procedures were performed in the lung area. The electrodes used were the condenser type, with a diameter of 13 cm. The method of placing is transverse on the chest and with a 3–4 cm distance between the electrodes and the chest surface. We used the oligothermal dose (medium heating) with the duration of the procedure of 10 min. The treatment course consisted of 10 treatments.

The algorithm used in the kinesitherapy was as follows: every day, two times per day the children performed three sets of 10 repetitions with a 2-min pause between each set. The program included was: increasing chest flexibility, improving posture, and correcting muscular imbalances of the respiratory and skeletal muscles through strengthening exercises for weak and lengthened dynamic muscles and relaxation of shortened static muscles, training in proper breathing [1, 5, 9–11, 12–14].

"Training in correct breathing" (**Figure 1**) aimed to correct the abnormal breathing pattern by slowing the respiratory rate at the expense of a more prolonged expiratory rate, reducing hyperventilation, using diaphragmatic-type breathing at rest (rather than abdominal or chest breathing), and using breathing through the nose (rather than the mouth) [15, 16]. "Training in correct breathing" was performed twice daily with three sets of 10 repetitions with a 2-min pause between each set [17].

Diaphragmatic breathing was facilitated by exteroceptive biofeedback (**Figure 1**). For this purpose, one hand was placed diaphragmatically. The maximal excursion was required when breathing in the diaphragmatic region rather than the abdominal or thoracic region. Diaphragmatic breathing was performed from functional residual capacity to maximal inspiratory lung volume with two consecutive interruptions while maintaining a 2:1 ratio of expiratory to inspiratory [17].

"Correction of respiratory muscle imbalance" (**Figure 2**) was performed two times daily with three sets of 10 repetitions with a pause of 2 min between each set [17]. Each repetition involved maximal inspiration through a wide open mouth (no resistance) from residual volume to total lung capacity in the lying down position [17]. To inhibit abdominal breathing, one hand was placed on the chest and no

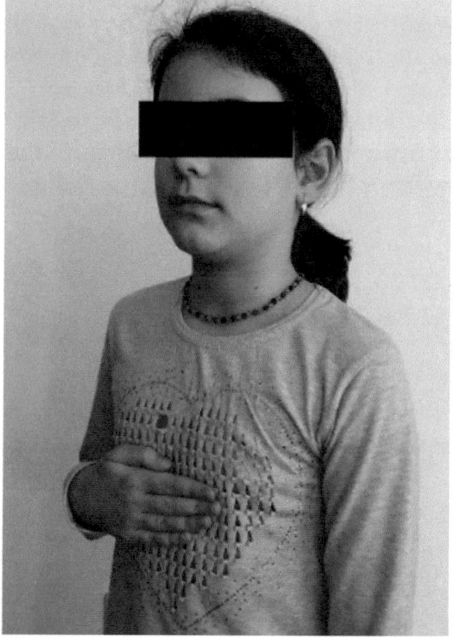

Figure 1.
Training in correct breathing.

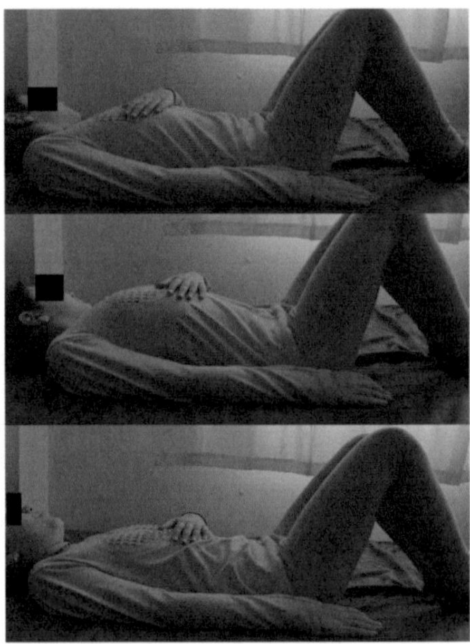

Figure 2.
Correction of respiratory muscle imbalance.

excursions were allowed in this area. For diaphragmatic respiration facilitation, the other hand was placed on the diaphragmatic area, and it was required that there be maximal excursions in this zone (**Figure 2**).

Expiration was performed through a narrowed slit of the mouth /between the lips/ (against resistance) within the functional residual capacity to avoid hyperventilation [17] (**Figure 2**). There were intervals of 60 seconds between these repetitions [17].

"Exercises to increase chest flexibility with postural improvement by correcting muscle imbalances" included chest extension in all planes [17, 18].

Horizontal thoracic flexibility (**Figure 3**) was exercised from a standing posture by the horizontal double arm and shoulder girdle swings in the opposite direction (initially with elbow joints flexed, then with elbow joints extended), which

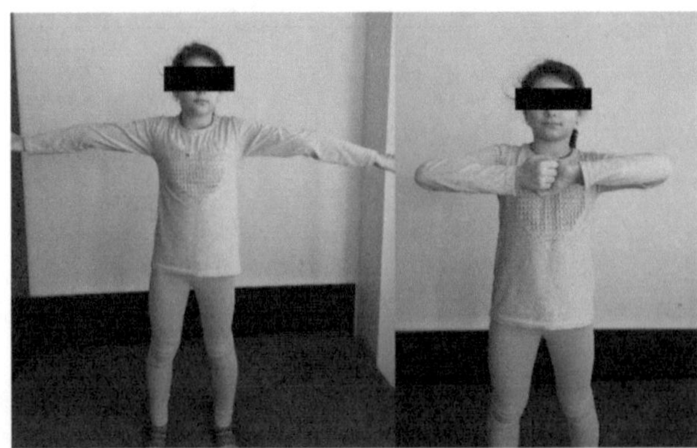

Figure 3.
Horizontal flexibility of the chest.

simultaneously relaxed the upper extremity and shoulder girdle adductors (predominantly static muscles) (**Figure 3**) [15–17].

Vertical thoracic flexibility (**Figure 4**) was exercised from a standing position by the vertical double arm and shoulder girdle swings in opposite directions (one arm

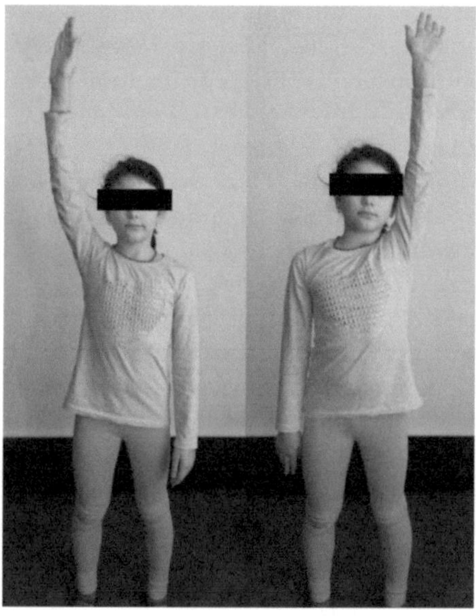

Figure 4.
Vertical flexibility of the chest.

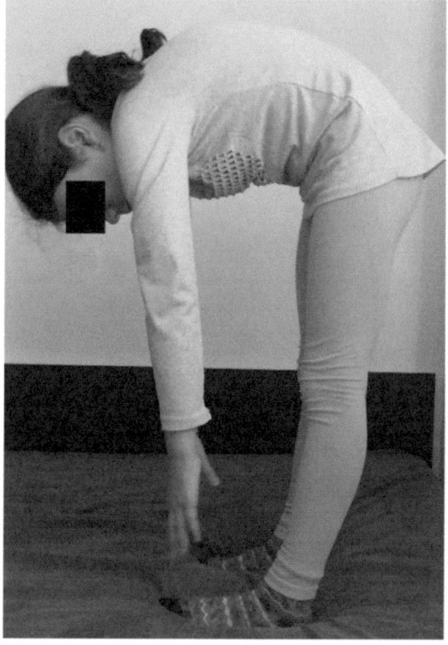

Figure 5.
Flexion sagittal flexibility of the chest.

cranially, the other caudally), which simultaneously relaxed the predominantly static upper extremity and shoulder girdle flexors [15–17].

Flexion sagittal thoracic flexibility (**Figure 5**) was exercised from standing to maximal forward and downward body tilt inducing total flexion of the entire spine, thoracic cage, and hip joints, which simultaneously relaxed the predominantly static extensors of the thoracic cage, trunk, and hip joints [15–17].

Extension sagittal thoracic flexibility (**Figure 6**) was exercised from standing to maximal backward and upward body tilt, inducing total extension of the entire spine, thorax, and hip joints, which simultaneously relaxed the predominantly static flexors of the thorax, trunk, and hip joints (**Figure 6**) [15–17].

Frontal thoracic flexibility (**Figure 7**) was exercised from a standing position by maximal bilateral lateroflexion of the body, inducing total lateroflexion of the entire spine and thorax, which simultaneously relaxed the predominantly static lateroflexors of the torso and thorax (**Figure 7**) [15–17].

Transversal rotational thoracic flexibility (**Figure 8**) was exercised from a standing posture by maximal bilateral body rotations inducing total rotation of the entire spine, the thorax, and hip joints, which simultaneously relaxed the predominantly static rotators of the trunk, thoracic cage, and the thorax (**Figure 8**) [15–17].

Three-dimensional flexibility and muscular balance of the thorax (**Figure 9**) and upper body in all planes were exercised from a standing position by full upper body circumduction circles alternating in both directions [15–17] (**Figure 9**).

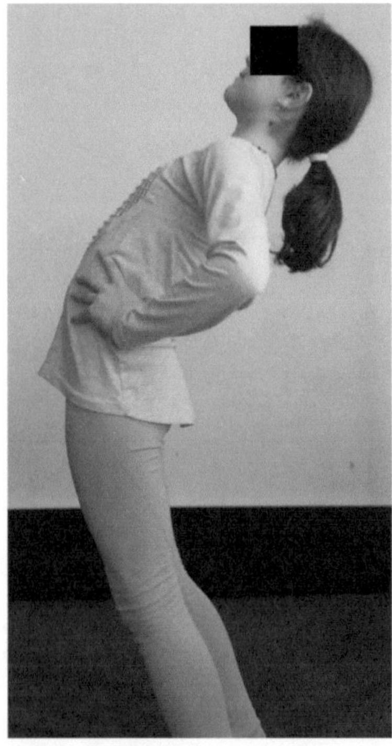

Figure 6.
Extensor sagittal flexibility of the chest.

DOI: http://dx.doi.org/10.5772/intechopen.109565

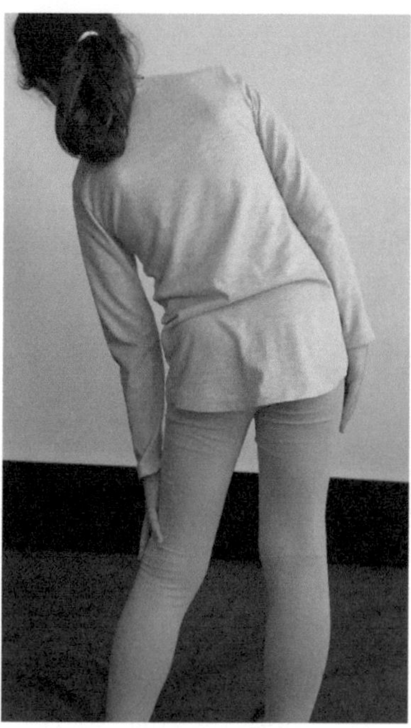

Figure 7.
Frontal flexibility of the chest.

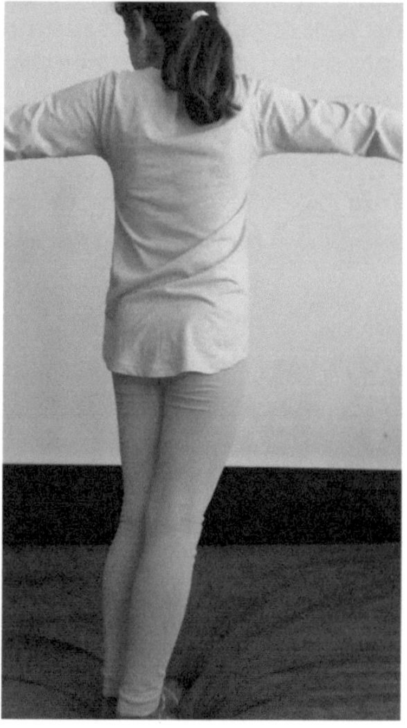

Figure 8.
Transverse rotational flexibility of the chest.

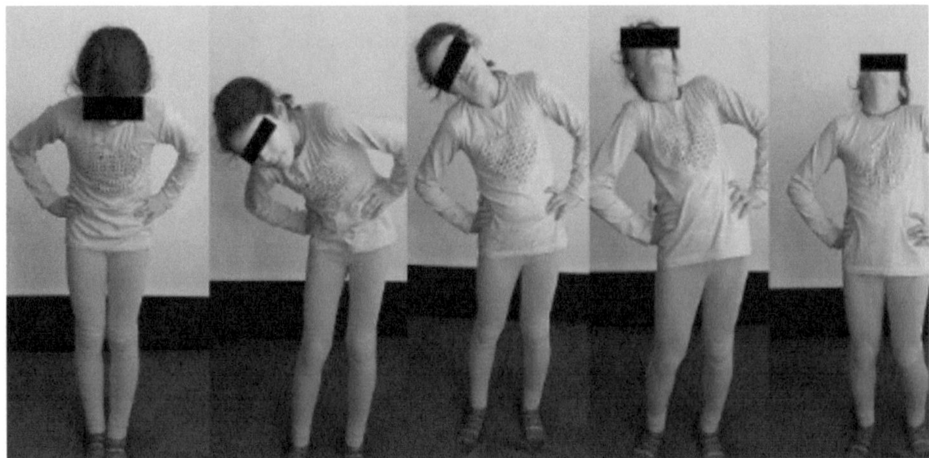

Figure 9.
Three-dimensional thoracic flexibility and muscle balance in all planes.

"Exercises to increase chest flexibility with postural improvement by correcting muscle imbalances" were performed two times every day with three sets of 10 repetitions with a 2-min break between each set [15–17]. The total duration of these exercises was 30 min daily (2 × 15 min).

At the beginning and end of the treatment course, the spirometric [18] and anthropometric [1, 5, 9, 11, 13, 14] parameters were recorded. The spirometric test was performed as follows—at each examination, we made three consecutive examinations with a computerized spirometer, and the best one was considered and recorded [18]. The anthropometric parameters were: age (g), weight (kg), height (cm), chest circumference at maximum inspiration, during a pause, and at maximum expiration, Erisman's index (chest circumference at pause—1/2 of height in cm), Brugsh's index (mean chest circumference divided by height in cm), Ott's test (spinal mobility in cm.), Tomayer's test (toe-to-floor distance in cm.), sagittal and frontal chest diameters and their ratio [5, 9, 11, 12].

Correlation analyses with post-hoc multiple linear regression tests were used to estimate the significance of the interaction between spirometric and anthropometric parameters, yielding significant real multiple regression formulas. We calculated the estimated spirometric parameters adjusted for all anthropometric parameters, based on these. These had higher statistical flexibility than the expected spirometric parameters calculated automatically by the computerized spirometer based on only three anthropometric parameters, which were age, weight, and height, which did not change over 10 days. We additionally included the ratios in percentages between the actual spirometric results and the expected spirometric parameters according to the obtained real regression formulas in the statistical analysis. For statistical analysis, a balanced MANOVA design with 2 × 2 levels of interaction was used, "before" in comparison with "after" treatment and the "physiotherapy" group in comparison with the "control" group. Bonferroni post-hoc multiple comparison tests were used to isolate the statistical clusters that were significantly different from the others.

3. Results

Concerning individual actual spirometric parameters and concerning ratios of actual versus computer-predicted spirometer parameters adjusted for age, weight, and height, there were no statistically significant MANOVA interactions ($P > 0.05$)

Based on the statistically significant multiple correlations ($P < 0.05$) between the actual forced expiratory volume in 1 second ("FEV1 Act1") and all anthropometric parameters, we calculated the following statistically significant multiple regression formula:

$$\begin{aligned}\text{"FEV1 Act1"} = {} & 4.14 + (0.0156^{*} \mathit{Age}) + (0.0189^{*}\,\text{Height}) + (0.0260^{*}\,\text{Weight}) \\ & + (0.0790^{*}\,\text{chest circumference } \mathit{at} \text{ maximum inspiratory}) \\ & - (0.0796^{*}\,\text{chest circumference } \mathit{at} \text{ maximum expiratory}) \\ & + (0.00435^{*}\,\text{chest circumference } \mathit{at} \text{ pause}) - (0.329^{*}\,\text{Brugsh's index}) \\ & - (0.000605^{*}\,\text{Erisman's index}) - (0.0233^{*}\,\text{Tomayer's test}) \\ & - (0.0682^{*}\,\mathit{Ott}\text{'s test}) + (0.198^{*}\,\text{sagittal chest size}) \\ & - (0.188^{*}\,\text{frontal chest size}) - (4.37^{*}\,\text{sagittal / frontal chest size ratio}).\end{aligned}$$

We applied this real formula to calculate the expected "FEV1 Pred1 formula" adjusted for all anthropometric parameters. We subjected the ratio between actual and expected forced expiratory capacity in 1 second according to this formula ("FEV1% Act1/Pred formula") to statistical MANOVA analysis with Bonferroni's post-hoc multiple comparison tests.

In comparison with the results after the 10-day course therapy with the combination of kinesitherapy and ultrahigh-frequency current and before the 10-day course, there was a significant increase in "FEV1% Act1/Pre formula" in the "physiotherapy" group, which was treated with the combination of kinesitherapy and ultrahigh-frequency current ($P < 0.05$), and "control" group (without kinesitherapy and ultrahigh-frequency current) ($P < 0.05$), but the "physiotherapy" group showed a

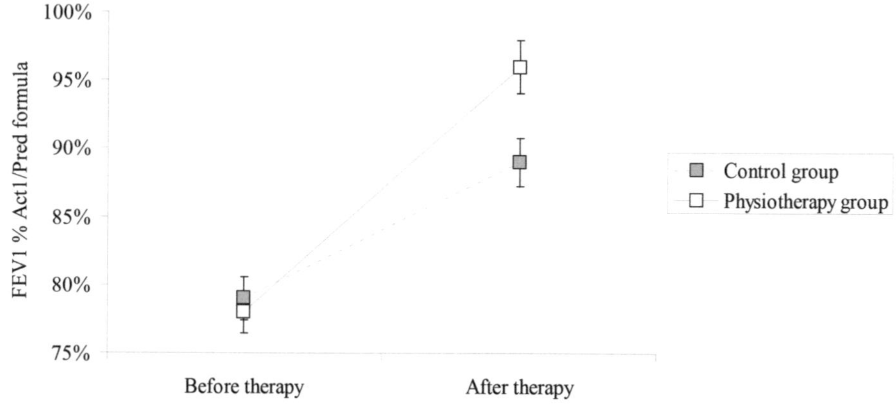

Figure 10.
The ratio between actual and expected forced expiratory volume in 1 second ("FEV1% Act1/Pre formula", adjusted for all anthropometric parameters), recorded before 10 days of treatment and after 10 days of treatment in the "physiotherapy" group (treated with the combination of kinesitherapy and ultrahigh-frequency current) and "control" group (without kinesitherapy and ultrahigh-frequency current).

statistically significantly higher value of this parameter compared with the "control" group after treatment (P < 0.05) (**Figure 10**).

We found out that the results of other spirometric parameters were similar when adjusted for all anthropometric parameters—chest circumference at maximum inspiration, during a pause, and at maximum expiration, Erisman's index (chest circumference at pause—1/2 of height in cm.), Brugsh's index (mean chest circumference divided by height in cm.), Ott's test (spinal mobility in cm.), Tomayer's test (toe-to-floor distance in cm.), sagittal and frontal chest diameters and their ratio.

4. Discussion

The actual spirometric parameters and the ratios of actual to computer-predicted spirometric parameters were insufficiently sensitive to reach statistically significant differences at the 10-day follow-up. The estimated spirometric parameters calculated by the computerized spirometer were based only on inert anthropometric measurements (age, height, and weight), and because of that, they could not verify improvement after the 10-day period. On the other side, the other anthropometric parameters showed sufficient flexibility and sensitivity over the 10-day follow-up.

Because we found in both groups an improvement after the 10-day treatment course in terms of the percentage ratios between actual and expected spirometric parameters, adjusted for all anthropometric parameters, this confirms the therapeutic effect of pharmacotherapy and rehabilitation with the combination of kinesitherapy and ultrahigh-frequency current in children with asthma.

But on the other side, the combination of kinesitherapy and ultrahigh-frequency current was found to have a better effect than pharmacotherapy in children with asthma, as the improvement after treatment was significantly greater in the "physiotherapy" group compared to the "control" group.

5. Conclusions

The combination of kinesitherapy and ultrahigh-frequency current has a significant therapeutic effect in a 10-day treatment of children with bronchial asthma, superior to that of pharmacotherapy.

Conflict of interest

The authors declare no conflict of interest.

Author details

Vyara Dimitrova*, Assen Aleksiev and Penka Perenovska
Medical University of Sofia, Clinic of Physical Medicine and Rehabilitation, Alexandrovska University Hospital, Sofia, Bulgaria

*Address all correspondence to: vtdimitrova@medfac.mu-sofia.bg

References

[1] Global Initiative for Asthma GINA. Global Strategy for Asthma Management and Prevention. United States: Medical Communications Resources; 2019

[2] Ivanova З, Veleva N, Glogovska P, Popova T, Ivanov Y. Cost of hospital treatment of patients with bronchial asthma. Medinfo. 2014;**2014**:12

[3] NHLNI Guideline. Bethesda, MD, USA: National Heart, Lung and Blood Institute; 2007

[4] Bojkov BM. Bronchial asthma - clinic and treatment. Medinfo. 2009;**2009**:12

[5] Cherniack NS, Altose MD, Homma I. Rehabilitation of the Patient with Respiratory Disease. USA: McGraw-Hill Companies; 1999

[6] Petrov D. Treatment and Rehabilitation of Bronchial Asthma. Sofia: Med. Phisk; 1991

[7] Perenovska P. Asthma in childhood. MedInfo. 2015;**2015**:2

[8] Yurukova V. Asthma in childhood. Medinfo. 2015;**2015**:8

[9] Goodgold J. Rehabilitation Medicine. St. Louis: C. V. Mosby Company; 1988

[10] Joschtel B, Gomersall SR, Tweedy S, Petsky H, Chang AB, Trost SG. Effects of exercise training on physical and psychosocial health in children with chronic respiratory disease: A systematic review and meta-analysis. BMJ Open Sport & Exercise Medicine. 2018;**4**(1):e000409

[11] Morgan M, Singh S. Practical Pulmonary Rehabilitation. London, UK: Chapman and Hall Medical; 1997

[12] Skalsky A. Pediatric Rehabilitation. Physical Medicine and Rehabilitation Clinic1s. Philadelphia: Elsevier Health Sciences; 2015

[13] Barker NJ, Jones M, O, Connell NE, Everard ML. Breathing exercises for dysfunctional breathing/ hyperventilation syndrome in children. The Cochrane Database of Systematic Reviews. 2013;**2013**(12):CD010376

[14] Del Giacco SR, Firinu D, Bjermer L, Carlsen KH. Exercise and asthma: An overview. European Clinical Respiratory Journal. 2015;**2**:27984

[15] Macedo TM, Freitas DA, Chaves GS, Holloway EA, Mendonca KM. Breathing exercises for children with asthma. The Cochrane Database of Systematic Reviews. 2016;**4**:CD011017

[16] Thomas M, Bruton A. Breathing exercises for asthma. Breathe. 2014;**10**(4):312-322

[17] Paiva DN, Assmann LB, Bordin DF, Gass R, Jost RT, Bernardo-Filho M, et al. Inspiratory muscle training with threshold or incentive spirometry: Which is the most effective? Revista Portuguesa de Pneumologia (English Edition). 2015;**21**(2):76-81

[18] Jat KR. Spirometry in children. Primary Care Respiratory Journal: Journal of the General Practice Airways Group. 2013;**22**(2):221-229

Chapter 4

Advancements in Endobronchial Ultrasound

Latrice Johnson and Clauden Louis

Abstract

Endobronchial ultrasound (EBUS) is a diagnostic procedure that allows for the diagnosis and staging of lung cancer and other lung-related diseases such as tuberculosis, sarcoidosis, and sarcoma. The radial probe for the EBUS device was first introduced to visualize the inside of the lungs and airway structures, and identify the extent of tumor invasion in the airway and surrounding lymph nodes. The EBUS transbronchial needle aspiration (TBNA) is an acceptable first test in the pretreatment staging of lung cancer to appropriately understand the prognosis for curative therapies. In the future, EBUS is likely to become widely available and accessible to patients, given its low cost and minimal risk of complications compared to other diagnostic and therapeutic procedures. The development of more advanced EBUS technologies, such as radial EBUS, virtual bronchoscopy, fluorescence-guided bronchoscopy, and artificial intelligence will allow for improved visualization of the lungs and adequate lymph node yield, leading to more accurate diagnoses and better treatment outcomes. In conclusion, the future of EBUS modalities combined with the additions of bronchoscopic advances is expected to further improve the accuracy and precision of the procedure while limiting morbidity, and complications, and improving clinical workflow availability in the outpatient setting.

Keywords: endobronchial ultrasound (EBUS), diagnostic imaging, bronchoscopy, endoscopic ultrasonography (EUS), electromagnetic navigational bronchoscopy (ENB), tumor sampling

1. Introduction

Bronchoscopy is a procedure by which physicians examine a patient's tracheobronchial tree. Generally, a bronchoscopy is conducted by traversing the vocal cords with the bronchoscope instrument through a patient's nasal, oral, or tracheal orifice. The most common type of bronchoscopy is that which utilizes a flexible bronchoscope. Certain conditions may arise that may require a different type of bronchoscopy such as rigid bronchoscopy in cases such as hemoptysis or obstructing lesions, or adjuncts such as endobronchial ultrasound (EBUS) or electromagnetic navigation bronchoscopy (ENB). In this chapter we will discuss the various types of bronchoscopies, adjunctions, indications, contraindications and procedural steps.

2. Flexible bronchoscopy

The flexible bronchoscope is one of the most widely utilized modalities for diagnosis and treatment of bronchopulmonary diseases due to its ability to reach distal airways, ease of use, and low risk procedural state in some cases only requiring mild to moderate sedation [1]. The outer diameter of the scope is anywhere between 2.2–6 mm, while the inner (working) diameter of the scope is between 1 and 2.2 mm [2]. The flexible bronchoscopy can be used for both diagnostic and therapeutic purposes. Indications for diagnostic purposes include refractory symptoms such as chronic cough, small volume hemoptysis, stridor, or pulmonary infections. Other diagnostic indications include unresolved pneumonia, interstitial lung disease, masses located in the lung, endobronchial or mediastinal, and chemical or thermal injury to the airways. Therapeutic indications for flexible bronchoscopy include tumor debulking, balloon dilation in benign central airway obstruction, abscess drainage, aspiration of cyst as well as airway stenting. Flexible bronchoscopy has a reported death rate of 0–0.04% in greater than 68,000 procedures, making it relatively safe. Major complications are equally infrequent with less than 1% of cases and if they occur could include respiratory distress, arrhythmias, cardiopulmonary arrest, major bleeding, and pneumothorax. This procedure is contraindicated in those that have preexisting arrhythmias and those who are hemodynamically unstable. This procedure also may be performed with moderate sedation which could cause an increase in heart rate that may induce ischemia in a small number of patients.

3. Rigid bronchoscopy

Rigid bronchoscopy is one of the oldest medical procedures in the thoracic field, however, use of this modality has declined with the introduction and ever increasing use of flexible bronchoscopy [2]. It actually has been recorded that the first use of this bronchoscope was in 1898 for the removal of a pork bone from the airways. Rigid bronchoscopy utility remains in the armamentarium of pulmonologist and thoracic surgeons given many of its benefits such as ability to both ventilate and stent open airways similar to that of an endotracheal tube but the opportunity to diagnose independently or simultaneously providing conduit for flexible bronchoscopy. The diameter of the scope measures from 3 to 18 mm for the outer scope while the inner (working) diameter of the scope is between 2 and 16 mm, making it larger than the flexible bronchoscope. In the setting of foreign body obstruction, the large diameter of the scope permits rigid bronchoscopy to remain advantageous for safe extraction compared to other modalities. Other therapeutic indications include management of malignant and benign central airway obstruction (CAO), and most importantly the management of massive hemoptysis. Due to large amounts of blood volume that can be lost in massive hemoptysis, a patient may develop asphyxia and hypoxia, leading to a life-threatening event. The rigid bronchoscope is used to stent an airway open, while providing therapeutic modalities to debride, debulk, or coagulate or irrigatethe airways for intraluminal patency.

Overall the rigid bronchoscopy is a life-saving therapy indicated for patients who have tacheobrnchial obstruction with inability to reliably ventilate. Potential complications include, injury to upper airway structures during intubation, hypoxia and hypercarbia, bleeding, and airway perforation. The most common symptoms reported after the procedure include a sore throat and neck pain.

	Flexible bronchoscopy	Rigid bronchoscopy
Diagnostic indications	Evaluation of: • Non-resolving pneumonia. • Ventilator-associated infections. • Diffuse lung disease. • Atypical chronic interstitial lung disease. • Parenchymal nodules or masses. • Confirmation of endotracheal tube position.	• Extraction of foreign bodies. • Evaluation of airway control during hemorrhage. • Airway stenosis. • Evaluation of the airway for tracheal resection. • Collection of large specimens for lung biopsies. • Examination of the subglottic airway in the neonatal population.
Therapeutic indications	• Placement of self-expandable airway stents. • Hemostasis of centrally located bleeding lesions. • Abscess drainage. • Use of ablative technique modalities.	• Management of bronchopulmonary hemorrhage. • Management of central airway obstruction (CAO) (both malignant and benign). • Placement of airway silicone stents. • Use of ablative technique modalities.

Table 1.
Indications for flexible bronchoscopy vs. rigid bronchoscopy.

The most common contraindications for this procedure are associated with the general anesthesia administered to the patient rather than the scope. Patients with very high oxygen requirements and those with high levels of positive end-expiratory pressure (PEEP) would typically not undergo this type of procedure. However, if the patient has CAO, and all other methods of oxygenation and ventilation have failed, rigid bronchoscopy would be performed to treat the patient's airways. Hypercoagulable states, cardiac conditions, facial trauma, neuromuscular conditions that can be worsened by anesthesia, and factors associated with atlantoaxial subluxation and instability should all be considered prior to this procedure (**Table 1**).

4. Endobronchial ultrasound (EBUS)

Endobronchial ultrasound (EBUS) is a procedure that combines the flexibility of a flexible bronchoscopy with a probe that specifically provides an angulated ultrasound image. The radial probe for the EBUS device was first introduced to visualize the inside of the lung's airway structures, and to identify the extent of tumor invasion in the central airway and the surrounding lymph nodes. EBUS is now routinely paired with the transbronchial needle aspiration (TBNA) procedure acquiring biopsies in a lesser invasive modality. EBUS transbronchial needle aspiration (TBNA) is an acceptable first diagnostic modality in the identification and pretreatment staging of lung cancer to appropriately understand the prognosis for curative therapies [3].

4.1 Physics

There are two types of EBUS probes: the radial catheter probe (RP-EBUS) and the convex probe EBUS (CP-EBUS). The RP-EBUS uses a thin catheter that contains a small probe and is passed through the working channel of the bronchoscope.

The probe rotates 360 degrees and captures ultrasound images of the lung parenchyma and the target lesion. This probe does not allow real-time needle biopsy; instead it is able to precisely locate pulmonary nodules or masses based on differences in echogenicity between normal lung tissue and other lesions [4]. RP-EBUS is a useful tool for lesions that are less than 2 cm or those commonly found in the smaller branches of the airway. The Convex-probe EBUS (CP-EBUS) has a linear ultrasound probe and an instrument channel on the tip of a bronchoscope, enabling an angulated needle biopsy under real-time ultrasound guidance [5]. The ultrasound mechanism utilizes high-frequency sound waves to create images of internal structures. The transducer within the device at the top of the bronchoscope, sends and receives ultrasound waves of the surrounding tissue and organs. The frequency of the sound waves used in EBUS are typically between 5 and 15 megahertz (MHz) with higher frequencies providing better resolution however superficial and in contradistinction, lower frequencies penetrating deeper however with lower resolution. Utilizing optimal depth and resolution, EBUS provides excellent visualization of structures adjacent to the airways, including lymph nodes and blood vessels, and for guiding biopsies of these structures. Based entirely on density and stiffness, EBUS ultrasound waves distinguish varying tissues while allowing less invasive specimen biopsy methodology for further testing. The thin CP-EBUS has improved accessibility to peripheral bronchi with excellent operability and is capable of sampling lobar and segmental lymph nodes using the aspiration needle.

5. Comparison of other techniques for tumor sampling

Surgical resection is traditionally the gold standard for obtaining mediastinal lymph node biopsy samples as well as curing early-stage lung cancer. Surgery can be performed with the traditional open approach (ex: thoracotomy) or by a minimally invasive approach. Video-assisted thoracoscopy (VATS) is a minimally invasive approach that is the preferred approach for surgical resection [6]. However, the needle techniques tend to be less expensive, less invasive, and have a smaller risk of complications when compared to surgical methods. Techniques for biopsy include previously mentionedEBUS-TBNA, Endoscopic Ultrasonography (EUS), mediastinoscopy, and Video-Assisted Thoracoscopic Surgery (VATS).

5.1 Endoscopic ultrasonography (EUS)

The EUS equipment consists of an ultrasound processor connected to an echoendoscope, with an ultrasound transducer attached at the distal tip of the instrument. The endoscope in return is connected to a standard video processor, permitting the endoscopic visualization [7]. This allows for simultaneous endoscopic and ultrasound imaging. EUS can use both a radial scope or linear scope to stage lung cancer in the mediastinum. However, radial scopes are most commonly used to stage lung cancer, while the linear scope is used for targeted EUS–fine-needle aspiration (FNA). EUS staging of lung cancer almost always requires FNA of lymph nodes in order to achieve greater accuracy. EUS can identify lymph nodes in the posterior and inferior mediastinum.

An advantage of EUS is that it can detect metastatic disease to subdiaphragmatic sites such as left adrenal, celiac lymph nodes, and liver. EUS-FNA is performed through the esophagus which presents as a limitation because ultrasonic rays cannot penetrate air-filled structures. This means the EUS-FNA cannot visualize or detect areas immediately anterior to the trachea [8].

5.2 Indications EUS versus EBUS

Patients that present with enlarged lymph nodes in the mediastinum on imaging should proceed to have an EUS or EBUS performed as the next step in the staging procedure [8].

Endobronchial ultrasound (EBUS) and endoscopic ultrasound (EUS) are two different procedures that use ultrasound imaging to visualize structures within the body. While they share some similarities, they have different indications and applications. The choice of EUS or EBUS is dependent on the location of the enlarged lymph node. Patients with enlarged lymph nodes in the posterior inferior mediastinum or subcarinal area are recommended to undergo EUS as the first staging procedure. Whereas patients with anterior, superior, or paratracheal lymphadenopathy may benefit from EBUS as the first staging test [8].

EBUS is performed through a bronchoscope and is used to visualize structures within the airways and lungs, including mediastinal and hilar lymph nodes. EBUS is primarily used for the diagnosis and staging of lung cancer, as well as for the evaluation of mediastinal lymphadenopathy. On the other hand, EUS is performed through an endoscope and is used to visualize structures within the gastrointestinal tract and adjacent organs, including the pancreas, liver, and lymph nodes. EUS is primarily used for the evaluation of gastrointestinal and pancreatic diseases, as well as for the diagnosis and staging of pancreatic cancer. While both EBUS and EUS use ultrasound imaging to visualize structures within the body, they have different areas of focus and applications. EBUS is more focused on the lungs and airways, while EUS is more focused on the gastrointestinal tract and adjacent organs. The choice of procedure depends on the specific clinical situation and the structures that need to be evaluated.

In general, EUS is most appropriate for evaluation of the posterior inferior mediastinum, whereas EBUS is better for the lymph nodes in the anterior superior mediastinum.

5.3 Medianstinoscopy

Mediastinoscopy is a surgical procedure that uses a mediastinoscope to examine the mediastinum— the space in the thoracic cavity between the lungs. In this procedure, the surgeon makes a horizontal cut 1 cm above the sternal notch to develop an anterior plane along the trachea. The surgeon then inserts the mediastinoscope and is able to sample and biopsy paratracheal and hilar lymph nodes. This procedure is useful for tissue sampling, mediastinal lymph node biopsy, and TNM staging. Mediastinoscopy has a high sensitivity (>80%) and specificity (100%) in the staging of lung cancer [9]. It can be classified into 2 different procedures: Cervical mediastinoscopy and Anterior mediastinotomy.

Cervical mediastinoscopy provides access to the pre-tracheal, paratracheal, and anterior subcarinal lymph nodes. However, it has limited access to the inferior and posterior mediastinum and the aortopulmonary window [8]. Anterior mediastinotomy is a procedure that allows for dissection of the aortopulmonary lymph nodes. Complications associated with this surgical procedure include pneumothorax, bleeding, nerve injury, and transient ischemia. The safety of the mediastinoscopy procedure versus EBUS are

Evaluation of sarcoidosis:	EBUS can be used to diagnose and evaluate the extent of sarcoidosis, a multisystem inflammatory disease that often involves the lungs and mediastinal lymph nodes.
Identification of tracheobronchial lesions:	EBUS can also be used to identify lesions or masses within the tracheobronchial tree, such as tumors or foreign bodies.
Treatment of obstructive lung diseases:	EBUS can be used therapeutically to relieve obstruction in the airways caused by conditions such as lung cancer, granulomas, or lymphoma.
Diagnosis and staging of lung cancer	Indications for EBUS include diagnosis and staging of lung cancer via sampling of central tumors, endobronchial specimen, mediastinal or hilar lymph nodes.
Distinguishing between benign and malignant lymph nodes	Etiologies of lymphadenopathy for which investigative efforts may be necessary include distinguishing between benign and malignant lymph nodes and guide biopsy for further testing. EBUS-TBNA is reported to have a sensitivity of 85–100%, a specificity of 100% and an accuracy of over 96% in distinguishing benign from malignant mediastinal lymph nodes in patients with lung cancer [8].

Table 2.
Indications for EBUS.

comparable with a mean cost of EBUS that is less costly ($P < 0.001$) and an associated lower risk of complications when performed as isolated procedures (Verdial et al).

5.4 Video-assisted thoracoscopic surgery (VATS)

VATS is described as a "keyhole' surgery in which 3 small incisions are made to perform the procedure. A 10 mm incision is made posteriorly to allow for the insertion of instruments, an additional 10 mm incision is made to allow the video thoracoscope to look inside of the thorax, and lastly a 3–4 cm incision is made to pull out the resected lobe [6].

VATS can only examine one side of the mediastinum at a time, because one of the patient's lungs often needs to be collapsed after general anesthesia. When the left mediastinum is being studied, nodal stations 5 (subaortic) and 6 (para-aortic) can be accessed. When the right mediastinum is being studied, nodal stations 2 and 4 (upper and lower paratracheal), station 7 (subcarinal) and stations 8 and 9 (para-esophageal and pulmonary ligament) can be accessed (**Table 2**) [8].

6. Role of EBUS in noncancer

EBUS-TBNA has proven to be useful in the detection of diseases such as sarcoidosis and tuberculosis (TB) which are classified by the presence of granulomas in thoracic tissue on biopsy.

6.1 Sarcoidosis

Sarcoidosis is an autoimmune disease that affects multiple organs and occurs mainly in African-Americans between the ages of 20–40. The cause of the disease is unknown, however, it can be diagnosed by the identification of clinical symptoms and lung biopsy. Many cases are asymptomatic (30 and 60%) and are diagnosed incidentally on a chest radiograph. When symptoms present they may include red painful bumps on the skin (erythema nodosum), arthritis, parotid enlargement and respiratory symptoms. On biopsy, sarcoidosis is classified by the presence of noncaseating granulomas [10]. EBUS-TBNA has been shown to be useful particularly for the diagnosis of stage I/II sarcoidosis in which the granulomas have spread to the lymph nodes resulting in hilar lymphadenopathy. The diagnostic yield of EBUS-TBNA for sarcoidosis ranges from 54 to 93%, which is higher than conventional transbronchial lung biopsy (TBLB) but still inferior to surgical biopsy. In order to improve the diagnostic accuracy of EBUS-TBNA, it is recommended to pair it with the EBUS-guided intranodal forceps biopsy (IFB) (EBUS-IFB) technique when sampling for tissue. This technique allows for a larger quantity of tissue collection that will contain larger amounts of DNA that is needed for extensive testing for suspected sarcoidosis.

The steps for the pairing of the procedures begin first with the puncture of an airway with a needle as part of the EBUS-TBNA procedure. Next, as part of the EBUS-IFB procedure, the miniforceps are inserted through the puncture site (with sonographic guidance) into the target lymph node to obtain biopsy samples [11]. The reported complication rates of this combined approach are higher than with EBUS-TBNA alone, but lower than with transbronchial or surgical biopsies.

6.2 Tuberculosis

Tuberculosis (TB) is an infection of the lungs caused by *Mycobacterium tuberculosis*. It is characterized by clinical symptoms such as blood-tinged sputum as well as caseating granulomas on biopsy. TB can also cause Benign mediastinal and hilar adenopathy. In a groundbreaking study conducted by Gupta et al., researchers reported that EBUS-TBNA has a high sensitivity (94%) and diagnostic accuracy (53%) in diagnosing TB [12]. The results of this study demonstrated EBUS-TBNA to be an effective and safe diagnostic procedure in patients with intrathoracic tuberculosis lymphadenitis (TBLA). Specific features on endobronchial ultrasound images that indicate tuberculosis lymphadenitis include heterogeneous echogenicity or coagulation necrosis of the lymph nodes. Differentiating tuberculosis from sarcoidosis during EBUS-TBNA is important due different treatment modalities and precautions surrounding tuberculosis [13].

6.3 Rapid on-site evaluation (ROSE) role

With the continued use of EBUS in the performance of lung biopsies for a large array of cancers and diseases, it is important to receive confirmation that the correct tissue sample is being biopsied. This can be accomplished with Rapid On-Site Evaluation (ROSE) to ensure sample adequacy and support a suspected diagnosis [14]. (ROSE) is a technique in which aspiration cytology samples are rapidly stained and screened for diagnostic material during the procedure. To make smears, the material from the needle is transferred onto a glass slide and smeared with a second slide to produce two direct smears (mirror slides). One smear is air-dried and stained immediately with a rapid Diff-Quik [DQ] stain and then evaluated on-site by the cytopathologist, and the second smear slide is fixed immediately in 95% alcohol for permanent cytologic examination using Papanicolaou stain. Inadequate results are samples that are reported as non-diagnostic, blood only, no tissue material, no nodal tissue, or scant tissue sampling [15].

The confirmation of a suspected diagnosis with ROSE provides guidance for subsequent samples and can result in reduced sampling, TBNA passes, and/or endobronchial biopsies. ROSE also reduces procedure time, exposure to anesthetic agents, and related complications that may occur due to the prolongation of the procedure [14]. These benefits can be seen across all indications for EBUS-TBNA, including sarcoidosis.

6.4 Possible complications

EBUS-TBNA is considered to be a safe procedure, with a reported incidence of 0.5% for infectious complications [16] and 0.05% risk for major complications in systematic reviews [8]. The risk of infection is very rare but increases dramatically in cases with target lesions of necrosis seen on chest CT. Necrosis typically occurs due to injuries, infection, or ischemia, and this provides an environment for decreased bacterial clearance leading to an increased risk of infection. The risk of infection also increases when EBUS-TBNA is combined with EUS-B-FNA. Oral and esophageal bacteria can be transported into the mediastinum during the passing of the needle in EUS-B-FNA [16]. Major complications of EBUS-TBNA include pneumothorax and respiratory failure requiring ventilation [8]. Recently additional complications related to needle breakage during the EBUS-TBNA procedure have been reported [17]. Needle breakage is rare; however, inhaling or swallowing a broken needle tip has the potential to cause serious complications to the patient.

6.5 Hybrid procedures

The outlook of EBUS as a less invasive diagnostic modality looks bright as it is expected to become an even more essential tool in the diagnosis and treatment of lung cancer and other lung diseases as it is combined with additional technologies such as navigational platforms and robotics. The development of newer and more advanced EBUS technologies, such as radial EBUS and virtual bronchoscopy, will allow for improved visualization of the lungs and adequate lymph node yield, leading to more accurate diagnoses and better treatment outcomes for lung cancer and other lung diseases.

6.6 Electromagnetic navigational bronchoscopy (ENB)

Electromagnetic navigational bronchoscopy (ENB) is a minimally invasive procedure that uses advanced imaging technology and navigation systems to guide interventionalists, thoracic surgeons, and bronchoscopists through the airways of the lungs to specific locations identified on cross-sectional imaging where possible tumors exist [18]. This technology allows for the diagnosis and treatment of lung cancer and other lung diseases with greater accuracy and precision than traditional bronchoscopy methods and the ability to access nodules and masses up to near the edge of pleural using nearby small bronchi.

A disadvantage of this procedure is that it can only be performed after obtaining a dedicated CT scan. This additional factor increases the patient's exposure to radiation and cost of treatment for the scan and software when compared to CT-guided biopsy. However, there are fewer complications when compared to a CT-guided biopsy including a pneumothorax rate as low as 1% [18]. ENB is indicated in the evaluation of peripheral pulmonary diseases, however it can also be used for evaluation of mediastinal lymphadenopathy, and is superior to the conventional TBNA [18].

7. Emerging bronchoscopy technologies

New and emerging technologies utilizing EBUS technologies are expected to further improve the accuracy and precision of the procedure as they are combined with 3D generated models utilizing virtual bronchoscopy from cross-sectional image rendering, fluorescence-guided bronchoscopy, and artificial intelligence.

7.1 Virtual bronchoscopy

As a new modality with great promise that is still evolving, virtual bronchoscopy is a technology that utilizes computed tomography (CT) images to create a 3D rendering model of the airways. This technology allows for the visualization of the airways in a way that is similar to traditional bronchoscopy, without the use of an actual bronchoscope as a non-invasive modality that can guide the utility of EBUS positioning to access distal samples.

7.2 Fluorescence-guided bronchoscopy

Fluorescence-guided bronchoscopy is a technology that utilizes fluorescent dyes to highlight abnormal tissue during the time of bronchoscopy. This modality allows for the detection of early-stage lung cancer and other lung diseases, and can improve the accuracy of biopsy and other diagnostic procedures. Combined with CT imaging and aided by EBUS tissue sampling detection of clinically occult neoplasms as well as symptomatic tumors are feasible [19].

7.3 Robotic bronchoscopy

Robotic bronchoscopy is a technological advancement that combines the precision and degrees of freedom of a robotic arm to control the steering of a bronchoscope. This technology allows for much greater flexibility and accuracy during bronchoscopy, and can improve the safety of the procedure for patients. Artificial intelligence (AI) is expected to play a major role in the diagnostic future of bronchoscopic modalities. AI-based systems can be used to analyze images and data from bronchoscopy procedures, helping to improve the accuracy of diagnosis and treatment [16].

7.4 Possible complications

EBUS-TBNA is considered to be a safe procedure, with a reported incidence of 0.5% for infectious complications [17] and 0.05% risk for major complications in systematic reviews [8]. The risk of infection is very rare but increases dramatically in cases with target lesions of necrosis seen on chest CT. Necrosis typically occurs due to injuries, infection, or ischemia, and this provides an environment for decreased bacterial clearance leading to an increased risk of infection. The risk of infection also increases when EBUS-TBNA is combined with EUS-B-FNA. Oral and esophageal bacteria can be transported into the mediastinum during the passing of the needle in EUS-B-FNA [17]. Major complications of EBUS-TBNA include pneumothorax and respiratory failure requiring ventilation [8]. Recently additional complications related to needle breakage during the EBUS-TBNA procedure have been reported [20]. Needle breakage is rare; however, inhaling or swallowing a broken needle tip has the potential to cause serious complications to the patient.

7.5 Unique case report

Unique case reports have described the use of vascular endobronchial ultrasound (VEBUS) in visualizing the location and characteristics of thromboembolic disease within the peripheral artery, such as chronic thromboembolic pulmonary hypertension (CTEPH). Characteristics identified on the convex probe EBUS include: thickening of the interlobar PA wall, an intraluminal fibrous web, and an intraluminal thrombus. The ability of EBUS to be able to visualize the location/ extent of disease is important for treatment outcomes for the patient. Limitations of VEBUS are due to the size of the EBUS probe which prevents the evaluation of vasculature beyond the branch point of the lobar PAs [18].

8. Conclusion

In conclusion, bronchoscopies are very important in the field of respiratory medicine. This procedure allows us to diagnose and treat a plethora of diseases, cancers, and conditions that may be life saving for the patient. The rigid bronchoscopy was the first technique used in the field and has become an important therapy for treating major hemorrhage. As medicine has continued to evolve, the use of the flexible has become very common and many use it for diagnostic purposes. The next major advance was the invention of the Endobronchial ultrasound (EBUS).

EBUS-TBNA is a widely used and accepted first diagnostic modality in the identification and pretreatment staging of lung cancer and other lung diseases. The concurrent use of ROSE in these procedures helps to increase accuracy and safety. As the indications for EBUS use continue to expand, EBUS is expected to play an even larger role in the diagnosis and treatment of lung cancer and diseases. The development of newer and more advanced EBUS technologies, such as radial EBUS and virtual bronchoscopy, will allow for improved visualization of the lungs and adequate lymph node yield, leading to more accurate diagnoses and better treatment outcomes. Additionally, EBUS is likely to become more widely available and accessible to patients, given the low-cost and with minimal risk of complications compared to other diagnostic and therapeutic procedures.

Furthermore, EBUS can be used for the diagnosis of other lung diseases as well, such as tuberculosis, sarcoidosis, and sarcoma, as the technology of both imaging and EBUS improves diagnostic yield is feasible at earlier disease states thus improving the chances of recovery.

The future of EBUS modalities combined with the additions of bronchoscopic advances is expected to further improve the accuracy and precision of the procedure while limiting morbidity, complications, and improved clinical workflow availability in the outpatient setting. These developments will help to improve patient outcomes, reduce recovery times, and make lung related diagnostics more accessible to patients around the world.

Author details

Latrice Johnson[1] and Clauden Louis[2*]

1 Howard University College of Medicine, Washington, DC, United States

2 Cardiothoracic and Vascular Surgery, BayCare Medical System, Florida, United States

*Address all correspondence to: claudenlouis@gmail.com

References

[1] Casal RF, Ost DE, Eapen GA. Flexible bronchoscopy. Clinics in Chest Medicine. 2013;**34**(3):341-352. DOI: 10.1016/j.ccm.2013.03.001

[2] Diaz-Mendoza J, Peralta AR, Debiane L, Simoff MJ. Rigid bronchoscopy. Seminars in Respiratory and Critical Care Medicine. 2018;**39**(6):674-684. DOI: 10.1055/s-0038-1676647

[3] Fielding D, Kurimoto N. Endobronchial ultrasound-guided transbronchial needle aspiration for diagnosis and staging of lung cancer. Clinics in Chest Medicine. 2018;**39**(1):111-123. DOI: 10.1016/j.ccm.2017.11.012

[4] JacomelliM,DemarzoSE,CardosoPFG, Palomino ALM, Figueiredo VR. Radial-probe EBUS for the diagnosis of peripheral pulmonary lesions. Journal Brasileiro de Pneumologia. 2016;**42**(4):248-253. DOI: 10.1590/S1806-37562015000000079

[5] Takahiro N, Kazuhiro Y, Taiki F, Ichiro Y. Recent advances in endobronchial ultrasound-guided transbronchial needle aspiration. Respiratory Investigation. 2016;**54**(4):230-236. DOI: 10.1016/j.resinv.2016.02.002

[6] Sihoe ADL. Video-assisted thoracoscopic surgery as the gold standard for lung cancer surgery. Respirology. 2020;**25**(S2):49-60. DOI: 10.1111/resp.13920

[7] Rossi G, Petrone MC, Arcidiacono PG. A narrative review of the role of endoscopic ultrasound (EUS) in lung cancer staging. Media. 2021;**5**:3. DOI: 10.21037/med-20-51

[8] Lankarani A, Wallace MB. Endoscopic ultrasonography/fine-needle aspiration and endobronchial ultrasonography/fine-needle aspiration for lung cancer staging. Gastrointestinal Endoscopy Clinics of North America. 2012;**22**(2):207-219. DOI: 10.1016/j.giec.2012.04.005

[9] McNally PA, Arthur ME. Mediastinoscopy. In: The National Library of Medicine: National Center for Biotechnology Information. StatPearls Publishing; 2023. Available from: http://www.ncbi.nlm.nih.gov/books/NBK534863/ [Accessed: April 12, 2023]

[10] Bokhari SRA, Zulfiqar H, Mansur A. Sarcoidosis. In: The National Library of Medicine: National Center for Biotechnology Information. StatPearls [Internet]. Treasure Island (FL): StatPearls Publishing; 2023. Available from: https://www.ncbi.nlm.nih.gov/books/NBK430687/ [Accessed: Junuary 25, 2023]

[11] Agrawal A, Ghori U, Chaddha U, Murgu S. Combined EBUS-IFB and EBUS-TBNA vs EBUS-TBNA alone for intrathoracic adenopathy: A meta-analysis. The Annals of Thoracic Surgery. 2022;**114**(1):340-348. DOI: 10.1016/j.athoracsur.2020.12.049

[12] Gupta N, Muthu V, Agarwal R, Dhooria S. Role of EBUS-TBNA in the diagnosis of tuberculosis and sarcoidosis. Journal of Cytology. 2019;**36**(2):128-130. DOI: 10.4103/JOC.JOC_150_18

[13] Ye W, Zhang R, Xu X, Liu Y, Ying K. Diagnostic efficacy and safety of endobronchial ultrasound-guided transbronchial needle aspiration in intrathoracic tuberculosis. Journal of Ultrasound in Medicine.

2015;**34**(9):1645-1650. DOI: 10.7863/ultra.15.14.06017

[14] Rokadia HK, Mehta A, Culver DA, et al. Rapid on-site evaluation in detection of granulomas in the mediastinal lymph nodes. Annals of the American Thoracic Society. 2016;**13**(6):850-855. DOI: 10.1513/AnnalsATS.201507-435OC

[15] Iliaz S, Caglayan B, Bulutay P, Armutlu A, Uzel I, Ozturk AB. Rapid on-site evaluation and final cytologic diagnoses correlation during endobronchial ultrasonography. Journal of Bronchology Intervention Pulmonology. 2022;**29**(3):191-197. DOI: 10.1097/LBR.0000000000000809

[16] Ghattas C, Channick RN, Wright CD, Vlahakes GJ, Channick C. Vascular endobronchial ultrasound in a patient with chronic thromboembolic pulmonary hypertension. Journal of Bronchology Intervention Pulmonology. 2021;**28**(2):e23. DOI: 10.1097/LBR.0000000000000713

[17] Kang N, Shin SH, Yoo H, et al. Infectious complications of EBUS-TBNA: A nested case-control study using 10-year registry data. Lung Cancer. 2021;**161**:1-8. DOI: 10.1016/j.lungcan.2021.08.016

[18] Paradis TJ, Dixon J, Tieu BH. The role of bronchoscopy in the diagnosis of airway disease. Journal of Thoracic Disease. 2016;**8**(12):3826-3837. DOI: 10.21037/jtd.2016.12.68

[19] Gilbert S, Luketich JD, Christie NA. Fluorescent bronchoscopy. Thoracic Surgery Clinics. 2004;**14**(1):71-77, viii. DOI: 10.1016/S1547-4127(04)00041-6. PMID: 15382310

[20] Uchimura K, Yamasaki K, Hirano Y, et al. The successful removal of a broken needle as an unusual complication of endobronchial ultrasound-guided transbronchial needle aspiration (EBUS-TBNA): A case report and literature review. Journal of UOEH. 2019;**41**(1):35-40. DOI: 10.7888/juoeh.41.35

Chapter 5

A Case of Endotracheal Tube Damage during Maxillomandibular Osteotomy Found by Bronchofiberscope

Michiharu Shimosaka

Abstract

We experienced a case of endotracheal tube damage during maxillomandibular osteotomy found by bronchofiberscope. The patient was a 22-year-old man, scheduled for maxillomandibular osteotomy under general anesthesia for the treatment of two jaws deformity. Tracheal intubation of Microcuff subglottic endotracheal tube (I.D.7.5 mm made by Halyard Health Care Inc.) was *via* the left nasal cavity. The surgery started from maxilla and became the maxillary transection approximately 50 min later. There was the indication of the ventilation gas leak from the operation after the maxillary transection, but we confirmed that, and there was no tube in the clear abnormal findings with bronchofiberscope. Because the positive pressure ventilation was possible, and the ventilation had no problem, we decided to resume surgery. After maxillary fixation was completed approximately 3 and a half hours later, and confirming with bronchofiberscope again, we confirmed an inflow of the blood in a tube and confirmed a tube laceration to around 4–5 cm from the nasal cavity entrance. We decided to conduct tube exchange. After the surgery, the cause of tube rupture was examined; it was then found that the tube was damaged by a bone chisel used during maxillary bone dissection. When there is doubt about a endotracheal tube damage, confirmation of the inner surface using a bronchofiberscope is useful, and it is important to grasp the case early.

Keywords: bronchofiberscope, tube rupture, nasotracheal intubation, maxillomandibular osteotomy, general anesthesia

1. Introduction

The damage of the endotracheal tube under general anesthesia causes respiratory failure. It is difficult to check the endotracheal tube in nasotracheal intubation; therefore, the use of the bronchofiberscope is effective.

We experienced a case of endotracheal tube damage that was discovered during maxillamandibular osteotomy by bronchofiberscope, which we have therefore reported.

I obtained consent from the patient concerned to report the present case.

2. Case subject

The patient was a 22-year-old male of 178 cm in height and weighing 85 kg. The patient was diagnosed with maxillamandibular deformity, and for the treatment, maxilla-mandibular osteotomy under general anesthesia was scheduled. There was no particular medical history or family history, and on preoperative examination, there were no particular findings observed.

3. Progress

There was no premedication administered, and the patient was admitted to a hospital in ambulatory condition. Anesthesia was introduced rapidly using remifentanil hydrochloride, propofol, and rocuronium bromide under oxygenation. For the tracheal tube, left-sided nasotracheal intubation was performed using a subglottic endotracheal tube® (Halyard Healthcare Inc.) with inner diameter of 7.5 mm. Cuff inflation was performed using a 5 ml syringe, airway pressure was 20 cm H_2O, and there was no air leak. Anesthesia was maintained with air pressure at 5 l/min, oxygen at 1 l/min, propofol at 4 mg/kg/h, and remifentanil hydrochloride at 0.2 μg/kg/min, and with additional administration of rocuronium bromide as needed.

Surgery was commenced from the upper jaw, and maxillary bone dissection was completed in approximately 50 minutes. After dissection, the surgeon identified a ventilation gas leak. As there was no clear displacement of the tube, endotracheal cuff insufficiency was suspected, and inflation was increased to 7 ml (cuff pressure of 27 cm H_2O). There was no decrease in cuff pressure, and a cuff abnormality was ruled out; however, the ventilation gas leak could not be stopped, and therefore, the tube lumen was verified by bronchofiberscope. However, there were no clear abnormal findings observed. Positive pressure ventilation was possible, and because there was no problem with the ventilation status, maxillary fixation was recommenced. Upon recommencement, ventilation gas leakage was verified again. Maxillary fusion was completed at approximately three and a half hours after verification of the initial leakage, and therefore, upon reverifying with a bronchofiberscope, blood inflow within the tube was confirmed, and tube damage at 4–5 cm from the nasal cavity inlet was confirmed (**Figure 1**). Thus, tube replacement was planned. While expanding the larynx, the damaged tube was removed, and orotracheal intubation was immediately performed. With orotracheal intubation, respiratory intubation was confirmed, a new tube (subglottic endotracheal tube® with inner diameter of 7.5 mm) was carefully inserted by left-sided nasotracheal intubation, and after passing through the nasal cavity, the orotracheal tube was removed, and intubation with the new tube was performed immediately.

After achieving nasotracheal intubation again, the ventilation gas leak disappeared. Thereafter, mandibular osteotomy was commenced and completed with an operative duration of 7 h and 59 min. Intubation upon returning to the wardroom was planned, and therefore, the patient was transferred to his ward under management by propofol at 2–4 mg/kg/h and fentanyl hydrochloride at 20 μg/h, and the duration of anesthesia after stable spontaneous respiration was 9 h and 54 min.

Upon searching for the cause of the tube damage postoperatively, we found that the damage was caused by the bone chisel used for maxillary bone dissection (**Figure 2**).

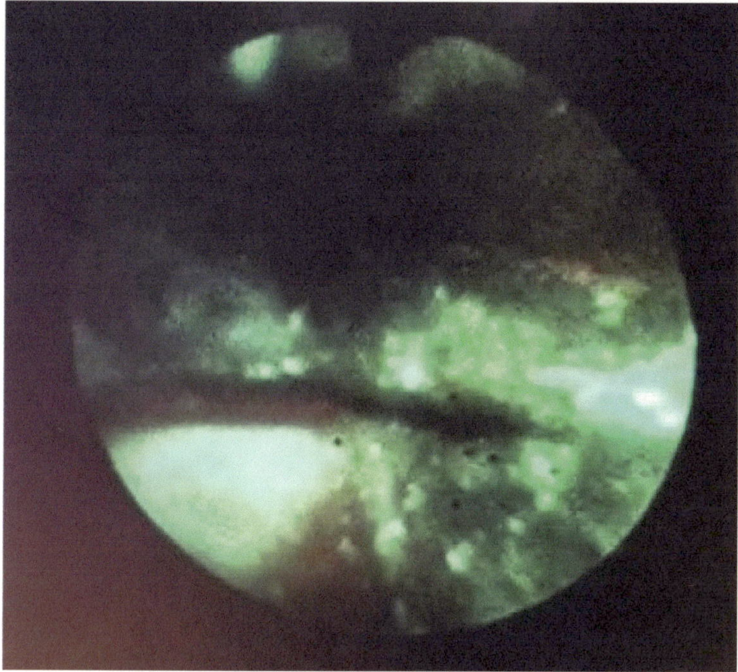

Figure 1.
Endotracheal tube damage found by bronchofiberscope.

4. Discussion

In this case, maxillary osteotomy was performed using the Le Fort I procedure. In the Le Fort procedure, osteotomy is performed from the piriform aperture to the lateral wall of the nasal cavity, anterior wall of the maxillary sinus, maxillary tuberosity, and the pterygomaxillary junction [1]. For this case, we used a reciprocating saw to dissect from the anterior wall to the lateral wall of the maxillary sinus, and used a bone chisel to dissect the junction between the maxilla and the sphenoid bone. In the postoperative verification, the blade shape of the bone chisel was consistent with the tube damage site, and therefore, the damage was judged to have been caused by the bone chisel. It was thought that the damage occurred when dissecting the junction between the maxilla and the sphenoid bone on the left side.

Although a cuff leak was initially suspected intraoperatively, it was judged that there was no decrease in cuff pressure and no cuff abnormality. Therefore, the inner surface of the tube was verified using a bronchofiberscope. With the initial verification, no clear damage could be confirmed, and there was no inflow of blood. The intubation tube that was used in the present case was a Microcuff subglottic endotracheal tube® (Halyard Healthcare Inc.) with an inner diameter of 7.5 mm; however, because suctioning can be performed above the cuff, the external diameter was 11.2 mm and the tube was thick overall. Consequently, time was required for the expansion of the damaged part and until blood inflow, which was thought to explain why there was no clear abnormality observed in the initial verification.

As a result, general anesthesia management was performed for approximately three and a half hours while the tube was damaged; however, in retrospection, it is possible that if the tube had been verified again, then the damage could have been detected

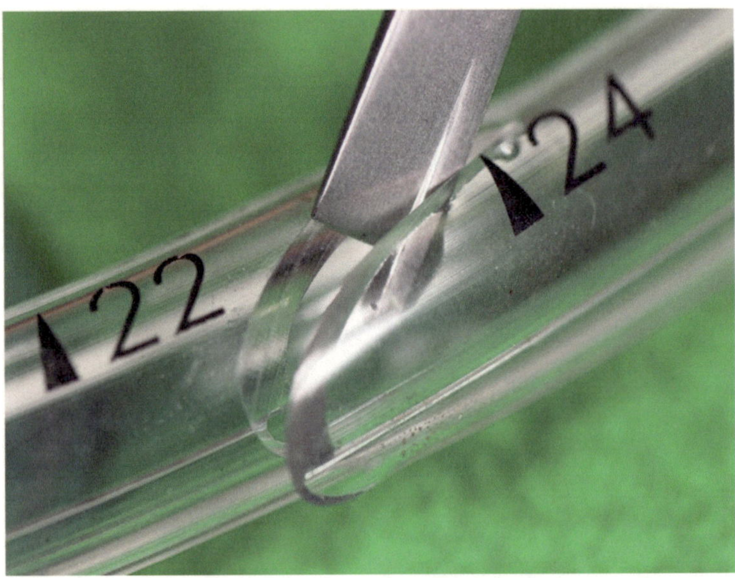

Figure 2.
The cause of tube rupture was damaged by a bone chisel used during maxilliary bone dissection.

earlier. When there is suspicion of endotracheal tube issues, it is important to identify the cause early, such as by verifying the inner surface of the tube once or twice per hour. In this although there was no inflow of blood into the trachea, a large volume of blood inflow as a result of tube damage has been reported [2], and a case of pulmonary collapse presenting with blood inflow has been reported [3], and therefore the risk of pulmonary complications is increased if verification of tube damage is delayed.

Several past reports can be found that describe similar endotracheal tube damage in Le Fort I osteotomy. One of such reports describes treatment by increasing the fraction of inspired oxygen and oxygen flow rate in the circuit [4], while another report describes tube damage repaired with tape and without removing the tube but rather pulling the tube out several centimeters [5]. However, in this case, because intubation upon returning to the wardroom was planned, and that the damage was verified at a point in time before commencing mandibular osteotomy, we chose to perform tube removal and repeat nasotracheal intubation.

With regard to re-intubation, the maxillary surgery was complete and normal expansion of the larynx was possible, and therefore, immediately after removing the damaged tube, orotracheal intubation was performed while performing respiratory management, after which a tube was carefully inserted into the left nasal cavity, and nasotracheal intubation was performed.

Repeat intubation was completed safely using video laryngoscopy and avoiding conventional laryngeal expansion has been reported [6], and it has also been reported that with actual video laryngoscopy, compared to the direct-viewing method, the visual field of the larynx is better, and tube insertion can thus be performed more rapidly and easily [7]. Therefore, the use of video laryngoscopy should probably be considered in situations where it is difficult to expand the larynx. Furthermore, for reliable re-intubation, the use of a tube exchanger should be kept in mind [8]; however, considering that it can be difficult to pass the tube through the nasal cavity immediately after maxillary osteotomy, as in this case, we avoided its usage.

5. Conclusions

We experienced a case in which endotracheal tube damage was detected during maxillamandibular osteotomy by bronchofiberscope. When endotracheal tube damage is suspected, it is useful to verify the inner surface of the tube using a bronchofiberscope, and it is important to identify the cause of the damage early.

Conflict of interest

The author declares no conflict of interest.

Author details

Michiharu Shimosaka
Department of Anesthesiology, School of Dentistry at Matsudo, Nihon University, Japan

*Address all correspondence to: shimosaka.michiharu@nihon-u.ac.jp

References

[1] Nakajima M. Standard surgical technique for jaw deformity. Japanese Journal of Oral and Maxillofacial Surgery. 2012;**58**(8):437-479

[2] Koyanagi N, Doi M, Mise K, Taniguchi S. Unexpected blood aspiration caused by endotracheal tube damage during operation. Journal of Japanese Dental Society of Anesthesiology. 2003;**31**(5):549-550

[3] Uno N, Terai T. Atelectasis caused by unexpected bleeding during induction of anesthesia: A case report. Journal of Japanese Dental Society of Anesthesiology. 2009;**37**(5):566-567

[4] Davies JR, Dyer PV. Preventing damage to the tracheal tube during maxillary osteotomy. Anaesthesia. 2003;**58**:914-915

[5] Takagi Y, Kurita T, Sato S. A case of endotracheal tube damage during maxillo-mandibular osteotomy. The Journal of Japan Society for Clinical Anesthesia. 2008;**28**(3):457-460

[6] Nakai K, Kitayama M, Niwa H, Hashiba E, Wada M, Hirota K. A case of successful tracheal tube exchange with airway scope® for tube damage during maxillo-mandibular osteotomy. Masui (Semi-official Organ of Japanese Society of Anesthesiologists). 2010;**59**:1315-1317

[7] Suzuki A, Toyama Y, Katsumi N, Kunisawa T, Sasaki R, Hirota K, et al. The Pentax-AWS ® rigid indirect video laryngoscope: Clinical assessment of performance in 320 cases. Anaesthesia. 2008;**63**:641-647

[8] Mort TC. Continuous airway access for the difficult extubation,: The efficacy of the airway exchange catheter. Anesthesia and Analgesia. 2007;**105**:1357-1362